These books have
Strong Start Team working in partnership
with Milk and You.
Strong Start are qualified Early Years
professionals commissioned by Public
Health to provide the universal part of the
Children's Centre Services offer for West
and North Northants
strongstartteam@westnorthants.gov.uk
07880136070
Milk&You are Public Health commissioned
breast feeding peer support volunteers
trained to offer guidance on infant feeding.
07949353423

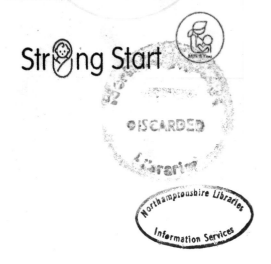

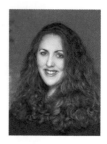

About the author

Sarah Ockwell-Smith specialises in the psychology and science of parenting, 'gentle parenting' and attachment theory, with a particular interest in child sleep. Sarah is famed for her gentle, science-rich, yet easy-to-read books, and her down-to-earth manner and ability to translate her vast knowledge of parenting science into easy-tounderstand language.

The mother of four school-aged children (three boys and one girl), Sarah lives with her family, cats and numerous ducks and chickens in a 350-year-old cottage in rural Essex, UK.

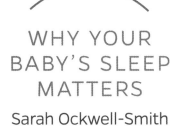

WHY YOUR BABY'S SLEEP MATTERS

Sarah Ockwell-Smith

Why Your Baby's Sleep Matters (Pinter & Martin Why It Matters: 1)

First published by Pinter & Martin Ltd 2016, reprinted 2018

© 2016 Sarah Ockwell-Smith

ISBN 978-1-78066-545-0
Also available as ebook

Pinter & Martin Why It Matters ISSN 2056-8657

Series editor: Susan Last
Index: Helen Bilton
Interior layout: Rebecca Longworth
Illustration on page 84: Jon Lander
Design: Blok Graphic, London
Cover illustration: Donna Olivia Smith

British Library Cataloguing-in-Publication Data
A catalogue record for this book is available from the British Library.

Set in Minion

Printed and bound in the EU by Hussar

This book has been printed on paper that is sourced and harvested from sustainable forests and is FSC accredited.

Pinter & Martin Ltd
6 Effra Parade
London SW2 1PS

pinterandmartin.com

Contents

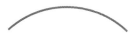

Author's Note

I want to begin this book with a few words about myself and my aims and hopes.

Fifteen years ago I became pregnant with my first baby. To my surprise mothering came to me easily and instinctively. To my great regret, however, I spent my first few years of motherhood sabotaging that instinct. Like the rest of my antenatal group, I read all the 'baby training' books that were in vogue at the time. I hated what I read in them, but felt that I wasn't qualified to question the 'experts'. I duly implemented their advice, backed by the opinions of the health professionals I came into contact with. The night I stood outside my son's bedroom door while he cried himself to sleep is one of the worst memories of my life, and the decision I regret the most. I've moved on from the guilt – after all, I thought my actions were in the best interest of my child – but the regret is ever-present.

When my other three children were born something in me woke up. I binned the books and started listening to my heart. They never cried themselves to sleep; I was there whenever they needed me and in some way I needed that too. I won't say that it was easy – it wasn't. It was bone-crunchingly tiring. I lived through five years of permanent exhaustion and sleep deprivation. There were many times I second-guessed my choice and times when I was tempted to sleep train, but every time I thought about giving up I remembered the night I stood outside of my son's room while he sobbed himself to sleep. That one memory kept me going and helped me to stay on a gentle path.

Since then I have worked with thousands of parents. All trying to manage the despair of sleep-deprived exhaustion, the desire to do what is best for the child, and the pull of their parental instincts. The most pertinent thing that I have learned is that the sleepless nights are always temporary. Even though it may feel like you will never have a full night's sleep again, I can promise that you will. This phase, as hard as it is, is transient. It will end. As much as you may wish it away now, there will be days and nights to come when you will wish that your baby was back in your arms again. The memories you will have for the rest of your life are worth so much more than a few extra hours of sleep. I've been there. I have worked with so many families that have been there. One day you too will be on the other side and you'll know just how much those early weeks and months mattered. You'll know how important your choices were and you will feel proud of them, not regretful.

This book isn't only written for parents. I hope that it will prove a valuable resource for health professionals and those who work with new parents. I strongly believe that the world is due a paradigm shift when it comes to the expectations and management of infant sleep, so thank you for reading this book and becoming one of the leaders of this movement. Your input is desperately needed.

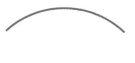

Introduction

A baby's cry is possibly the most unsettling, intolerable sound there is. For good reason. Babies cry to communicate to us that they need something. That may be a physical need such as hunger or thirst, discomfort or pain, or it may be a psychological need such as the need for comfort and human touch. All of these needs are equally valid.

When a baby cries, our instinctive motivation is to tend to it, whether the baby is ours or not. When we hear a crying baby our bodies respond; quickening our pulse and putting us on high alert. The sound is deliberately nerve-jangling and attention-grabbing. The same response is seen in all mammals, not just humans. We are hard-wired to find a baby's cry distressing, and we are hard-wired to respond. When we hear a crying baby responses programmed by our DNA drive us to pick the child up and offer comfort. This response is a protective mechanism for our species. If the human race is to survive, it is imperative that we protect our young.

These innate drives are not regulated by the clock. A baby's cry is just as serious at night as it is during the day. Needs do not decrease as the sun sets. A baby's physical and psychological needs exist no matter what the time. As adults our instincts do not diminish when our head hits the pillow. Why then has it become commonplace to ignore not only a baby's cry, but also their needs at night? This question perplexes many, including myself. When did we, as humans, sever ties with all of our mammalian relatives and decide that we would only listen to our intuition during daylight hours? That our parenting would be relegated to only 12 out of 24 hours? When you think of it like this, the fact that we ever ignore the cries of our young at night is ridiculous. We are supposedly the most intelligent species on planet Earth, but sometimes we certainly don't act like it!

The issue of 'night-time parenting' needs exploring and is crying out (no pun intended) for a change in our society's approach. Questions that we urgently need to ask include:

- Why does baby sleep matter?
- Is it possible to meet the needs of both baby and parent?
- What happens when we do not respond to a baby's physical and psychological needs?

In Chapter 1 we will look at these questions and investigate where it all went so wrong for *homo sapiens* when it comes to sleep. In chapters 2, 3 and 4 we will take some time to understand the biology of baby sleep, comparing and contrasting the sleep of infants with that of adults and the young of other species. It is important to start with an exploration of normal infant sleep, and that means how a breastfed baby sleeps – as breastfeeding is biologically normal for our species. We'll look at what happens to infant sleep when babies are fed the milk of another species too. Many believe that 'giving a bottle' will make a baby sleep for longer, but does the research agree? For most parents, baby sleep at night is the main source of anxiety, but daytime naps can also cause stress and worry, and for this reason Chapter 3 is solely devoted to the discussion of daytime naps. What does the science tell us they should really look like, and how do we commonly inhibit them?

Chapter 5 looks at the question of when night feeds become 'abnormal'. When is a baby too old to still need milk at night? Is there an age by which a child should be able to sleep through the night without food and drink? What would happen if parents *never* night weaned? Is feeding at night a 'bad habit'? Does it encourage babies to keep waking? These are important questions that many parents and others have strong opinions about, but what does the evidence say? It turns out that much of what we think we know about infant sleep is wrong.

Chapters 6 and 7 consider infant sleep from a historical and cultural perspective. How did we end up where we are now? Have we always struggled so much with sleep, or did our ancestors find night-time parenting easier? What, if anything, can we learn from them? Is baby sleep an issue worldwide, or something that is more problematic in certain parts of the world? Are our babies really the problem, or is our modern Western lifestyle to blame? Can we rely on the information and advice given to us by the media, experts and health professionals? These chapters are the ones that interest me the most. The idea that we have created our current predicament is uncomfortable to entertain, but important to explore.

Chapters 8 and 9 cover the uncomfortable topics of Sudden Infant Death Syndrome (SIDS), co-sleeping and bedsharing. These are three words that needn't go together, but sadly, through lack of understanding, commonly do. I aim to dissociate them once and for all.

Chapters 10 and 11 address some of the practicalities of

being a parent of a baby. Yes, baby sleep matters, but so does adult sleep. The key is finding a balance, where the needs of all members of the family are considered and – ideally – met. Exhaustion is a feeling all too common to new parents, and we are frequently reminded of how many hours of sleep we will lose in the first year of a baby's life. Chapter 10 discusses ways in which this exhaustion can be minimised.

'Is he good?' is a question guaranteed to solicit eye-rolling and sighing from any new parent. Often the question is followed by unsolicited sleep advice, from everyone from family members to strangers in the street. These suggestions are often well meant, but they can cause high levels of anxiety and doubt for parents. Chapter 11 therefore discusses ways in which parents can not only ward off, but cope with sleep advice, particularly when it is at odds with their chosen methods, or even worse, critical of them.

Finally, in my opinion, no parenting book is complete without stories from those who are the true experts in babies: parents themselves. Chapter 12 is packed with stories from those who have been there and know what it really feels like to be wrung out and at the end of their tether, and yet survive. I hope they will inspire you as they did me.

Baby sleep matters, for so many reasons. How we treat our babies in their early weeks and months can and does shape them for the rest of their lives. Those babies grow and in turn have dramatic effects on the lives of others, including their own children. Baby sleep, and the way adults cope with it, matters because it has a knock-on effect that ultimately affects the future of us all.

NB: This book is primarily concerned with the sleep of infants, which means babies up to the age of 12 months, although much of the information is relevant for older babies and toddlers too.

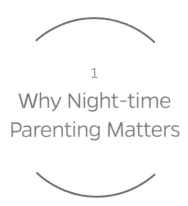

1

Why Night-time
Parenting Matters

The fact that 'night-time parenting' exists as a phrase shows that something is wrong with parenting in our society today. If a baby cries in the daytime, their cries will likely be responded to swiftly. At night-time, however, it is a different story. Thousands of babies will cry themselves to sleep tonight; thousands more will be left to cry alone when they wake in the middle of the night. Combined, the noise of all of the babies left to cry tonight would be deafening. A joint chorus of confusion, fear, loneliness, hunger and pain. Some may be left to cry for only a few minutes, while others will be left to cry until their voice becomes hoarse, their eyes sting and their tear-stained face swells before they finally succumb to sleep, not in sweet peaceful contentment, but from exhaustion and for self-preservation. Some babies will become so distressed, and will cry so lustily and for so long, that they will vomit. Some will give up crying as their parents stand unmoving at the nursery door, or sit stone-like and unresponsive on a chair a few feet away from the cot.

This is not a description of a television advertisement

raising awareness about cruelty to children: it is reality. A reality that will be played out in many, many homes tonight. Imagine the outrage if this behaviour occurred during daylight hours! Would such disregard for a baby's needs be acceptable during the daytime? The same professionals that recommend this style of sleep training at night preach the importance of connection, responsiveness, bonding and attachment during the day. The behaviour so many parents are advised to display during the night would often be classified as neglect during the day, by the very people who are recommending it. It is an ironic and disturbing dichotomy.

Why does night-time parenting matter? It matters because parenting is parenting, no matter whether it happens during the day or at night. There should be no difference in the way we respond to our children's needs based upon the clock. A need is a need whether it occurs at midday or midnight.

In the course of researching this book I asked some parents why they think night-time parenting matters. Quite a few replied with words to the effect of *'I don't understand what you mean? What is night-time parenting?'*. If all parents felt the same there would be no need for baby sleep books. It would be accepted that babies have needs 24 hours a day, and that a parent's role is to respond to them. After all, there are no working-time regulations when it comes to parenting, however much we might sometimes wish for them.

Here are some of the responses I received to my question, 'Why does night-time parenting matter?':

'A baby's needs don't stop when the sun goes down, if anything it's more important that the baby knows he can call us and we will come to help.'

'There is no magic age when babies suddenly no longer need

parental help at night. It's an unhappy truth for many, but it is true, despite what the expert books and websites want us to believe. Continuous broken sleep does make life hard, but it's only for a relatively short period of time and ultimately our babies will be better off when we keep parenting at night for as long as is necessary.'

'You commit to loving your baby well before they are born, that's 24/7, not just when it suits you.'

'Babies need sleep for their bodies and brains to grow. If my baby needs me to sleep with him and nurse him all night long then that's what he'll get. I want him to know he can count on me whenever he needs me, not just when it's convenient for me.'

'Nights are the hardest part of parenting, but I think maybe the most important. My child is an infant so won't remember these sleepless nights, but I try to remember that in twenty years I will give anything for one more night-time cuddle.'

'I don't see any difference between day and night when it comes to parenting, if she needs me, she needs me.'

'I just want my son to be happy, to feel loved, to trust his parents and to believe the world is a safe and happy place. I never could let my baby cry. I can't let my baby feel hurt without the comfort of his parents' arms.'

'I believe that the way I parent through the night will contribute to my son being a confident, loving and empathic person. So I will continue to be a responsive parent through the night until he no longer needs me.'

'Babies need care and love; responding to them is crucial, it doesn't matter what time it is or what others say. Being patient and empathic in the night results in a happy baby who feels safe.'

Is it possible to teach a baby to 'self-soothe'?

The idea behind almost all forms of baby sleep training is the teaching of 'self-soothing', or 'self-settling' skills. The presumption is that babies are born not knowing how to get themselves to sleep, and that if parents do not teach these vital life skills then they will be disadvantaging their child for life. A child not taught to 'self-soothe' will supposedly be a problematic sleeper, reliant on their parents at night forever more. Is this really true?

When I run baby sleep workshops I ask two simple questions of my audience. The first is: *'Can you, as an adult, self-soothe all of the time?'* Almost everyone will answer 'no' to this question. Certainly we all know adults with short tempers and low emotional intelligence.

Think about the last time you felt very scared, anxious, sad or angry. How did you manage to calm down? Your list may include any, or all, of the following: a cup of tea, alcohol, chatting with a cyber friend, chocolate, cuddling a loved one, crying, deep breathing, exercise, meditation, phoning a friend, self-talk, sex and turning on a light. There are probably many others I haven't mentioned. Now, how many of these can a baby do by itself, if it is lying in a cot alone? The answer is just one: crying.

If you were very scared, anxious, sad or angry and you began to cry, you might feel better after a few minutes because of the emotional release. Stopping crying at this point almost always involves other calming strategies, however, particularly 'self-talk'. You might think rationally about the situation and resolve to change, or perhaps accept it; perhaps you hypothesise about the best and the worst outcomes and how you could influence these. We know that babies aren't capable of this type of sophisticated thought. What would happen if you weren't able to regulate your own emotions and continued to cry? If a friend or relative was close by to hug you and talk to you, it would help significantly. They would act as an *external regulator* for your feelings. But what would happen if there was nobody to comfort you, and your crying was out of control and beyond your capacity to calm yourself? You would probably cry until you exhausted yourself. Perhaps you would cry yourself to sleep, or perhaps you would shut down a little and harden to the feelings inside of you in a form of self-preservation.

The second question I ask of my audience is: *'If you have a toddler, can they self-soothe?'* This question isn't normally answered in a conventional sense; it's usually met with laughter. Picture this: you make your toddler a drink in their favourite blue cup. Unbeknown to you, today they wanted the red cup. They have decided today that red is their favourite colour and they must only drink out of red receptacles. You hand your toddler their drink, in the blue cup, which they throw on the floor. Then they throw themselves on the floor too, crying like a wounded animal. They wanted the red cup, and only the red cup will do. Will the toddler employ techniques to regulate their emotions? Will they engage in self-talk, and remind themselves that it doesn't matter what colour the cup is? They have water, they are thirsty and the red cup holds the water perfectly well. They may be disappointed that the cup is blue, but it is still a cup and the water contained in it will still quench their thirst. Tomorrow they might get the red cup and all will be right with the world. Of course not. Toddlers tantrum because they cannot regulate the big emotions that arise in them. Their brains and thought processes are not yet fully connected and sophisticated enough for this sort of rational, critical and hypothetical self-talk. Toddlers don't tantrum because they are naughty, they do so because their brains do not allow them to calm themselves down.

So if adults can't always self-soothe, and toddlers can't self-soothe at all, why do we expect babies to be able to do it? What really happens when we systematically ignore a baby's cry, which signals an unmet need? Can they talk themselves through the loneliness, fear or anxiety they are feeling? Can they resolve their feelings of hunger or thirst? Can they do a spot of mindfulness or deep breathing to calm down? I know that this may sound far-fetched if you have never thought about a baby's sleep in this way before. But in reality it is no more far-fetched than the idea that leaving a baby to cry for a set period of time will teach them to be able to control their own emotions by 'self-soothing'.

The development of emotional self-regulation

Many psychologists believe[1] that the development of emotional regulation depends on the presence of certain cognitive processes, such as a good level of language, memory and something known as 'means-end' behaviour. Means-end behaviour implies a certain amount of theorising on the child's part. They start with a goal in mind and actively seek to perform actions that can lead to the goal. In the case of 'self-soothing', this would imply that the baby can understand that they want to be calm, and think about ways to reach a state of calmness using the objects and abilities available to them at the time. This complex chain of cognitive processes is clearly beyond the capability of babies.

The prevalent psychological belief is that a child does not begin to take part in any *active* emotional regulation until at least their second year of life, with the main phase of emotional regulation development occurring between three and four years of age. Even then the child's capabilities will not be equivalent to those of an adult. This change in emotional control between age three and four is largely accounted for by the child's ability to suppress their most dominant response to a situation and replace it with another, more appropriate, response. In the case of a baby waking in the night, perhaps experiencing anxiety or loneliness, their dominant response would be to cry for parental attention. In order to control their emotions in other ways, such as finding comfort from a cuddly toy, the baby would have to consciously suppress the usual 'cry' response. Once again this is a behaviour that is beyond the capability of babies.

The neurological implications of ignoring a baby's needs at night

When an infant's needs are not met at night, the baby is at risk of long-term ill effects on their ability to handle stress and their emotions. These ill effects are mostly concerned with the development of brain structures relating to emotional regulation and control, including the hippocampus, amygdala and pre-frontal cortex. In addition, exposure to stress during infancy, due to a lack of parental response, can damage the baby's developing HPA-axis.

The HPA-axis regulates an individual's response to stress; the term describes the connections between the hypothalamus and the anterior lobe of the pituitary gland in the brain and the adrenal cortex at the top of the kidneys. In a complicated chain of events these organs ultimately result in the secretion of the stress hormone cortisol. Increased secretion of cortisol as a response to stress enables the body to enter into 'fight or flight' mode.

Research[2] suggests that a baby's HPA-axis is regulated by maternal behaviour, especially through feeding and touch, which help the baby to secrete oxytocin, which in turn acts to suppress the HPA-axis and thus the stress response. In contrast, being exposed to high levels of stress[3] can leave a baby at risk of developing a hyper-reactive HPA-axis, which may mean that they struggle with stress and emotional regulation for the rest of their life.

Some argue that sleep training is not stressful for babies, but research[4] has demonstrated the negative effects of one common form of sleep training, controlled crying, on the baby's HPA-axis. Cortisol samples were taken from babies and their mothers during the process of controlled crying. As you might expect, levels of cortisol were high in both babies and mothers during the first few days of sleep training, correlated with the level of crying. What may come as a surprise is that the cortisol levels *remained elevated*, even when the babies stopped crying. The mothers, seeing that their babies were no longer crying, no longer experienced increased levels of stress, yet the silence did not indicate the absence of stress in the babies. So why did the babies stop crying? Their cortisol levels showed that they were not calm, or soothed: no 'self-soothing' had taken place. Why then were they no longer vocalising their distress?

The importance of this research, aside from raising important questions about the concept of self-soothing, lies in the *absence of comfort* by the mothers during the sleep training. We know that maternal presence helps to regulate a baby's HPA-axis and thus inhibit cortisol secretion. If the mothers had picked up their babies, instead of leaving them to cry alone in their cots, it is feasible to expect a reduction in the secretion of cortisol in both mother and baby. It can be strongly argued, therefore, that a baby crying in arms at night will not experience stress in the same way as a baby who is not in physical contact with a parent. It is not the *crying* that is the problem, rather it is the presence, or not, of a parent's comfort.

The true path to sleep independence

It is widely agreed that the ability to express and self-regulate emotions is a key component of psychological health. If asked, most parents would probably agree that they would like their child to grow into a confident adult, not afraid to share their feelings and capable of controlling their own urges. These are some of the key elements of happiness. Good emotional regulation skills are vital if an adult is to have peaceful and successful relationships with others, both personal and professional. Good emotional regulation skills allow adults to successfully resolve conflict, without resorting to verbal or physical violence. Good emotional regulation skills allow adults to express their emotions, rather than internalising them, where they may manifest as anxiety, depression, self-harm and eating disorders. Older children and adults with good emotional regulation skills find it easier to concentrate on their studies and career and work towards achieving their ambitions in life. Being able to regulate emotions doesn't mean not having feelings, or denying them – quite the contrary. It means the acceptance of feelings and the ability to work with them, rather than becoming overwhelmed by them.

The key question parents should ask themselves is *'How can I help my child to grow up to possess good emotional regulation skills?'*. When a child is capable of controlling their own emotions, only then are they truly able to 'self-soothe' or settle themselves when they are anything but calm. Cultivating 'emotional intelligence' is the easiest and most successful way of ensuring that children are able to sleep well independently. What does this look like in practice?

The general consensus in psychology is that children will grow to have good emotional regulation skills if their parents allow the child to express their feelings and, perhaps more importantly, validate them. This means that feelings are not dismissed because they may seem inconsequential or inconvenient to the adult. Feelings are not misunderstood and labelled as 'a habitual behaviour', or 'a manipulative behaviour', as a baby's attempts to communicate at night often are. Allowing expression and validating emotions in babies means *never ignoring their sole means of communication* – crying – day or night.

The more we respond to a baby or child's attempts to communicate their needs, the more confident they will be that their feelings will be heard and responded to by their parents. The more confident they become that their needs will be met, the more their bodies and psyche can develop the independence necessary for them to be able to calm themselves. This has been clearly illustrated by neuroscientific research[5] looking at changes in the infant brain in response to parental nurturing. Scientists have found that maternal nurturing during infancy leads to an increase in hippocampal volume in later childhood. This finding is of great importance, as the hippocampus is the area of the brain responsible for regulating emotions.

Further research[6,7] has found that there is a positive relationship between the way mothers help babies and toddlers to regulate their emotions, and the ability of the child to regulate their own emotions as they age. The more the mothers listen to and validate the child's emotions in infancy, and provide support and reassurance, the more the child is able to control their own emotions independently as they grow.

So why does night-time parenting matter? *Because it is the foundation of independence.* How a child is parented in their earliest months and years dictates how they will behave as they grow. What could be more important? The research is unequivocal. Self-soothing cannot be forced upon a baby, but behaving in an empathic, nurturing manner by meeting the baby's needs, day or night, is a sure-fire way to ensure that the child will truly be able to self-soothe when they are cognitively ready.

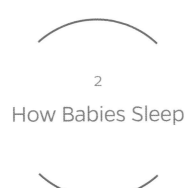

2

How Babies Sleep

Babies don't sleep like adults. So why do we expect them to? The uncomfortable truth is that when it comes to expectations of baby sleep, the problem almost always lies with our adult expectations, not our babies' biology. There are many ways in which baby sleep differs from adult sleep. Let's look at each in turn.

Babies have shorter, and more, sleep cycles

The phrase 'sleep through the night' is misleading. Babies don't sleep through the night, and neither do adults. In fact it is physically impossible for a human of any age to sleep through the night. No matter our age, we do not sleep in one long chunk. We do not simply go to sleep at night and wake in the morning. Each and every one of us moves through several cycles of sleep that as a whole make up 'a night's sleep'. An adult sleep cycle is around one and a half hours long. An average adult, getting seven to eight hours of sleep per night, will move through five different cycles of sleep each night. Each cycle of sleep will contain the two main phases of sleep: Rapid Eye Movement (REM) and non-Rapid Eye Movement (nREM).

REM sleep is characterised by a high level of activity in the brain and faster brain waves, but a virtual paralysis of muscles within the body. This sharp contrast has earned REM sleep the name 'paradoxical sleep'. This is the phase of dreams, and the eyes dart around beneath closed eyelids: hence the term 'Rapid Eye Movement'. REM sleep is also characterised by an irregular heart rate and rapid and irregular breathing. In contrast, nREM is the restorative phase of sleep. During this phase the body uses significantly less energy, as body temperature and blood pressure drop, brainwaves slow, muscles relax, eyes stop moving and the tissues of the body repair and restore themselves. nREM sleep is subdivided into a further three stages: N1, N2 and N3 (N3 is commonly known as delta sleep). Each of these levels of nREM sleep is progressively deeper and characterised by further slowing of brain waves. N1 is often described as a feeling of drowsiness or a light sleep, while N3 is deep sleep and considered the most restful of all of the phases. At each point it will be progressively harder to awaken the sleeping individual.

Each sleep cycle moves through the levels of sleep in turn:
N1 → N2 → N3 → REM → N1 (and so on)

Babies begin to sleep in cycles from roughly the 28th week of gestation.[1] Before this the brain activity of foetuses shows an erratic, immature electrical pattern. It is not until after week 36, however, that foetal sleep cycles are continuous and look more similar to those of adults. At birth a baby's sleep cycle lasts for around forty-five minutes, slowly increasing to nearer to sixty minutes at the end of the first year. These shorter sleep cycles mean that babies have roughly twice as many sleep cycles per night than adults, which in an average twelve-hour night of infant sleep could mean between twelve and sixteen different sleep cycles. If we remember that at the end of a sleep cycle a baby will return to a drowsy and possibly awake state, then this means that there may be up to sixteen occasions per night when they may wake and need parental assistance to go back to sleep.

Babies have more REM sleep

The difference in total length of sleep cycles is not the only difference between baby and adult sleep. The amount of REM and nREM sleep also differs greatly between babies and adults. A baby's sleep cycles begin to develop while they are still in utero. Initially the sleep is erratic with no real discernible pattern. As described above, patterns resembling sleep cycles begin to appear and mature between 28 and 36 weeks' gestation. At this stage most of the foetus's sleep is REM sleep. REM sleep is important for the development of the foetus's brain and related abilities, which explains why it is prevalent during this vital time of growth.

Once the baby is born, the need for the brain and body to develop and grow is just as pressing. The proportion of REM sleep therefore remains much higher than it is for adults. The lighter sleep experienced during REM sleep also acts as a protective mechanism against Sudden Infant Death Syndrome (SIDS) (see Chapter 9). Over the first year of life the amount of REM sleep experienced gradually decreases from 50 per cent of all sleep at birth,[2] to 40 per cent at four months, 30 per cent at six months and 25 per cent as the baby enters toddlerhood. An adult's sleep is composed of approximately 20 per cent REM and 80 per cent nREM.

It is important to understand the implications of this difference in REM and nREM ratio between babyhood and adulthood. Remembering that REM sleep is light and more easy to arouse from helps us to understand why babies wake more easily than adults in response to stimuli such as a change in sleeping place, or difference in temperature after falling asleep in the warm embrace of arms and being placed in the cold of a crib or cot. Furthermore, this additional REM sleep allows the baby to experience more dreams, and more nightmares. Any fear or anxiety from these can disturb the baby and cause them to wake and seek parental reassurance, even if the environment is unchanged and sleep-friendly.

Babies don't have established circadian rhythms, and we inhibit what they do have

Circadian rhythms are the 'internal body clock' that tell us whether it's time to sleep or time to be awake. The term comes from the Latin phrase '*circa diem*', which translates as 'around a day'. This continuous circular rhythm lasts for around 24 hours, based on our body's reaction to the presence or absence of daylight.

When our eyes are exposed to daylight, the photosensitive cells within them trigger an impulse via our optic nerve, situated at the back of the eye, which sends a signal to a region of the hypothalamus in the brain known as the suprachiasmatic nucleus (SCN). The SCN then signals to the pineal gland and other homeostatic areas in the hypothalamus to secrete the hormones cortisol and melatonin, as well as regulating body temperature.

During the day the presence of light, or more specifically short-wave (blue) light, initiates a chain reaction that concludes with the secretion of cortisol, which helps us to feel alert and awake. At night the absence of short-wave light triggers the secretion of melatonin and a lowered body temperature, which initiates sleep. Importantly, the presence of long-wave (red) light does not interfere with the release of melatonin in the same way that short-wave blue light does. This long-wave light is reminiscent of the natural lighting effects of a sunset or a burning fire or candle. The use of artificial, electric lights that emit blue light can override the natural cyclical rhythm and interfere with the secretion of melatonin. For optimal normal sleep, the environment must be free of artificial lighting during the evening and overnight. The light from energy-saving light bulbs, televisions, tablets and mobile phones is particularly disruptive when it comes to circadian rhythms, as they emit blue light. Other blue-coloured light sources, such as those commonly used in children's night lights and bedtime projectors, have the same effect.[3,4]

During pregnancy the foetus receives a certain amount of maternal cortisol and melatonin via the umbilical cord, in accordance with day and night-time. After birth the newborn infant loses this 'borrowed' circadian rhythm, but is yet to develop an established circadian rhythm of their own. For this reason newborns cannot 'tell night from day', and thus sleep erratically over a twenty-four hour period with no discernible night and day pattern. At around twelve to fourteen weeks of age the baby's circadian rhythm will begin to establish itself, but it does not reach full maturation, comparable to that of an adult, for some months.[5,6] There is no point trying to mark the difference between night and day in an attempt to 'teach' the baby when to sleep, if the necessary biological processes have not yet developed. Only time will bring the changes necessary for the baby to sleep more at night. Taking care over artificial lighting will not encourage the circadian rhythm to develop any sooner, but it will not inhibit any development that is taking place.

Babies' sleep is 'purer' than adults' sleep

It is ironic that so many baby sleep experts warn parents not to allow their babies to develop 'bad habits'. As adults we have far more negative sleep habits than any baby. Two of the most ingrained habits we have are late morning waking and ignoring our biological pre-programming to be active in the middle of the night.

As mammals, we 'should' rise in the morning in line with the sun. In most countries sunrise occurs between 4:30am in early summer and 7:30am in the very depths of winter. The average year-round sunrise sits at around 5:45am. If you visited a zoo you would find most of the diurnal (that is, not nocturnal) animals would be up and about with the rising of the sun. Meanwhile adult *homo sapiens* with blackout blinds and closed curtains continue to sleep long after sunrise. For their offspring, however, it is often a different story. Unaffected by the learned habits of their parents, human babies will respond to the rising levels of light in the same manner as their mammalian cousins. This is the normal biological response to the arrival of morning. We are all meant to be 'early wakers'. It is adults that have a 'late waking problem'. In time, through our behaviour and most likely the use of blackout fabric, our children will inherit our bad habits as they learn to override their innate instincts and biological processes. When that happens we no longer consider them to have an 'early waking problem'.

Similarly, if we could travel back through time to a couple of hundred years ago, before the invention of electric lights, we would also find the widespread pattern of another 'bad habit' in the making: polyphasic or segmented sleep. We would find that our ancestors did not sleep in one solid block of sleep all night; instead they commonly slept in two distinct segments, which they would refer to as 'the first sleep' and 'the second sleep'. The first sleep would usually commence after sunset and last for around four hours, followed by a period of being awake and active, commonly between one and two am. After this period of activity – which was coincidentally commonly recommended to be the best time to conceive a baby! – our ancestors would then take a second sleep until sunrise.[7] Since our babies do not yet know that it is no longer acceptable for humans to sleep in two segments, they are often wide awake between one and two am, and resist sleep for an hour or more until they begin their second sleep. It is not until they understand social norms that we can expect them to inherit our bad habit of ignoring thousands of years of normal human sleep biology and sleep in our abnormal, night-long pattern.

Babies need nutrition during the night

At the end of the first week of life a baby's stomach can hold a maximum of two ounces of milk. By the end of the first month, the maximum it can hold rises to five ounces. In many cases, however, the capacity is lower. The average capacity of an adult stomach is around thirty-five ounces.[8,9] Looking at these figures it is obvious why babies need to feed frequently! While many believe that babies do not need night feeds after a certain number of months, there is no evidence to suggest an arbitrary cut-off. As adults we often wake and take a sip of water or other liquid; why would babies not do the same?

Chapters 3 and 9 discuss the importance and impact of night feeds in far more detail.

Babies cannot 'self-soothe' or regulate their sleep environment

As adults our lives are fairly static, particularly when it comes to changes within our bodies. Babies, however, have many changes to contend with, including recovery from birth, reflux and other feeding-related issues, teething, developmental spurts and changes in abilities, such as the ability to roll, sit, crawl and 'pull up'. Psychological development, including separation anxiety and object permanence, introduces further change. In addition, part way through the first year babies transition to solid foods. All of these changes can understandably cause babies to become unsettled. Sleep can often regress and babies will tend to seek more external reassurance from their parents due to their inability to regulate their own internal or external environment. The first year in particular is rife with change. Just as a baby becomes comfortable with the way things are, their equilibrium is disturbed as they enter a new stage of development. With this in mind it seems naive to expect sleep to remain unchanged. Perhaps more naive is the commonly held expectation that sleep will continuously improve as the baby gets older.

How much sleep should babies really get?

This is an almost impossible question to answer, although it is often asked. The simplest response is 'as much as they need to', as sleep needs differ for each individual baby. Any *recommendations* given are just recommendations, and trustworthy sources will provide a rough guide rather than a fixed number of hours. Most recommendations about the length of time babies should sleep for, which often include suggested bedtimes and prescribe the length and number of naps, are not evidence-based. Many are based on personal opinion, and some authors are more educated than others.

Recent guidelines from the National Sleep Foundation[10] provide a broad range for the amount of sleep at each age. During the first three months anything between eleven and nineteen hours of total sleep per day may be acceptable. Between three and eleven months these figures change to a range between ten and eighteen hours. At twelve months between nine and sixteen hours of total sleep in a twenty-four hour period is indicated. What is not made explicitly clear is that these figures combine night-time and daytime sleep. A baby who sleeps for eleven hours at night at the age of three months may take only two very short naps, perhaps each totalling thirty minutes, but is still within the range of acceptability in terms of total sleep per twenty-four hour period. Similarly, a six-month-old taking two naps of one and a half hours each may only sleep at night for a total of seven hours, and will still fall within the normal range.

Recent research[11] has questioned the importance of paediatric sleep guidelines. Researchers from the Murdoch Children's Research Institute in Australia studied the sleep patterns of 4,000 children and concluded that associations between mental and physical health and well-being and sleep are overrated. The study found inconsistency between the amount of sleep a child had and their well-being levels and those of their parents, concluding that guidelines for specific amounts of sleep at each age may not be necessary or useful.

While researching this book I asked over 200 parents the question '*Before you had children, at what age did you think babies began to sleep through the night?*'. Their responses were as follows:

Less than three months: 22%
Between three and six months: 42%
Over six months: 8%
Over twelve months: 8%
I didn't know what to expect: 20%

These responses reflect the commonly-held expectation in our society that most babies should sleep through the night by six months of age. Research findings, however, paint a very different picture. At the age of three months research[12] has found that almost 47 per cent of babies wake *three to four times at night*. At six months of age research[13] has shown that 84 per cent of babies are still waking at night at least once. At twelve months of age research[14] has found that 50 per cent of babies still need parental help to get back to sleep when they wake in the night! These percentages are likely to be underestimated in most cases, as the great majority of research into infant sleep patterns relies on parent reporting of night-waking. Knowing that all babies wake at least once per hour, it is therefore likely that what the parents are actually reporting is when their babies *were crying for their attention* during the night. Research[15] shows that diary-keeping and parentally reported night-waking is an inaccurate measure for recording actual infant night waking. Using actigraphy, in which a sensor is worn by the baby to monitor movement, to measure night-waking proves that parents under-report the number of times their baby woke in the previous night. In other words, even if parents *believe* that their babies 'sleep through the night', they actually don't. What they are really saying is 'I do not need to go to my baby in the night when they wake'.

Once again we need to ask ourselves, '*Are baby sleep problems actually adult problems?*'. If evidence-based expectations of baby sleep were universally adopted, it would be easy for all to see that what is expected of baby sleep in our society today is unrealistic. Once our expectations are adjusted, it becomes clear that what many perceive as 'baby sleep problems' relate to babies that are sleeping perfectly normally.

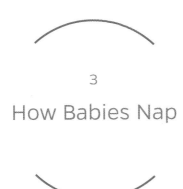

3

How Babies Nap

There is no doubt that daytime naps are a huge source of concern and stress for many parents. At any moment of any day there are parents walking, rocking and driving around in a frantic bid to get their baby to sleep for a daytime nap. Parents invest in blackout blinds, sleep shades and vibrating rockers and swings in order to lull their baby into a daytime slumber. The number and length of naps per day preoccupies many parents, and countless books about naptimes claim to have the 'right answer'. Let's look at what we actually know about naps.

Why babies need to nap

Scientists believe that babies nap for several different reasons. The most obvious reason is that the need for sleep accumulates more quickly during waking hours for babies than it does for adults. This means that for babies taking a nap is biologically necessary. Babies' extremely high levels of brain activity, due to the fast-growing size and connectivity of the brain, mean that they cannot tolerate long periods of time awake like older children and adults.

Research[1] has found that naps are an important way for babies to process their memories and to consolidate learning. Scientists believe that daytime naps help to strengthen a baby's memories during processing in the hippocampus and storage in the baby's long-term memory. This effect does not wane as the child grows; sleep is an important component in adult memory too. At a young age, however, the formulation and storage of memories is more critical to the way the baby makes sense of the world around them and develops new abilities. Importantly, the same research showed that this effect was gained after a nap time of only thirty minutes. Although naps are clearly important in infancy, the length of nap needed may not quite match the guidelines frequently given to parents.

Babies also nap during the day because of immature circadian rhythms. At birth a newborn does not know the difference between night and day and will sleep as much during the day as they do at night. As the baby grows and their circadian rhythm begins to develop this daytime sleep will naturally decrease over the first year of life. Circadian rhythms also impact on baby naps due to the homeostatic processes of different levels of alertness and sleep, which help the baby to regulate their breathing, heart rate and body temperature. Naps can therefore help to regulate the physical well-being of the baby's body. The baby's immature system means that they cannot tolerate long periods without the homeostatic regulation of sleep.

Research[2] has also shown how daytime naps help young children to regulate cortisol levels. Babies were shown to secrete cortisol shortly after waking from a morning or afternoon nap, but the same did not happen in the evening. The researchers therefore theorised that naps help to increase levels of alertness during the day, and also help babies to cope with any potential stressors they encounter.

How naps affect night-time sleep

For babies, the saying 'sleep breeds sleep' may well be true. If a baby's cues are followed during the day, and the parent allows the baby to sleep when they are tired and stay awake if they are not, then it is likely that they will be ready to sleep well at night. If a baby's cues are missed, perhaps through efforts to implement a parent-led daytime routine, or by undertaking too many daytime activities, there is a strong likelihood that the baby's cortisol levels will rise and they will become overtired or overstimulated towards the end of the day. This can result in difficulty in both falling asleep and staying asleep at night.

In toddlers, however, the evidence suggests a different correlation. Research[4] indicates that after the age of two daytime napping results in later night sleep onset, reduced sleep quality and less overall sleep at night. Once again the key lies in following the lead of the baby or child, rather than the expectations and recommendations of experts.

Where babies nap

Around the world the most common location for a baby to nap is in close physical proximity to the mother, or other family member. Often the baby is carried in a sling or baby carrier. In most cases this carrier is a single piece of cloth tied around the body, such as a Mexican rebozo. Many African mothers carry their babies in a simple piece of fabric throughout the day while they get on with their work. In Western society babywearing is becoming more popular, but there remains a stigma about 'creating bad habits' and 'carrying the baby too much'. Prevalent Western sleep advice centres on the importance of the baby sleeping alone in their crib or cot for daytime naps, and also focusses heavily on building a daytime nap schedule. Many babies, however, will fall asleep more easily and sleep for longer during the day if they are carried. Research[5] indicates that babies who are carried during the day cry significantly less than those who are not. A calm baby is a baby who is likely to find it easier to go to sleep and stay asleep. There can be no bad habits if the needs of the baby are simply being met. There are no demands for more from the baby. As the baby grows their need for maternal proximity during sleep will naturally lessen, and the child will eventually outgrow the need to be held or carried for naps. Until then it makes no sense to avoid meeting their needs in the present for fear of creating problems in the future.

Many mothers choose to co-nap with their babies. The shared daytime sleep provides a valuable way for the mother to catch up on sleep which may have been lost at night. Not only does sharing a nap with a baby help the baby to feel more secure, often resulting in a much longer nap, but it also helps the mother to regain some strength and energy for the rest of the day and coming night. This mutually beneficial sleep-sharing is a common practice in other cultures.

Interestingly, research[6] has found that keeping babies close for daytime naps may also help to reduce the risk of Sudden Infant Death Syndrome (SIDS). Most SIDS cases happen when the baby is unobserved by the parents. This is especially true of daytime naps, as the research found that 75 per cent of daytime SIDS occurred when the baby was sleeping alone in a different room from their parents.

The napping environment

Many parents in Western society make one big mistake when it comes to daytime naps. The common use of blackout blinds and sleep shades for car seats, prams and buggies during the day is at odds with the human circadian rhythm. The human body responds to the presence or absence of light by secreting either cortisol or melatonin. These chemicals tell the body whether it is time to be awake, or to sleep. For our circadian rhythms to function optimally we need to observe natural levels of lighting, both at night and during the day. We know that artificial lighting at night can disturb sleep,[7] which more parents are beginning to take note of. What is less well known, however, is the negative effect of making the daytime artificially dark.

Under-exposure to light in the daytime has been shown to have negative effects on circadian rhythms.[8] Exposing babies to *more* light in the daytime has a positive effect on circadian rhythm and thus night-time sleep.[9] While blackout blinds may be useful at night, they should not be used in the daytime. The same is true of the sleep shades commonly used on car seats, prams and buggies. Just as products that create artificial light during the night negatively affect sleep, so too do products that create artificial darkness during the daytime. The developing circadian rhythms of babies need as much natural light and exposure to darkness as possible. Anything that interferes with this should be avoided, even if it may appear to make the days easier. A price will be paid at night.

What to expect by age

Many parents are keen to know exactly how long their baby should be napping for at a particular age. Websites and books advise them how many naps their baby should have per day, and how long each nap should last for. Often this advice is displayed in easy reference tables, divided neatly by age in months. Unfortunately these tables are based upon nothing more than personal opinion. There has actually been very little research into infant nap requirements. There is no such thing as 'evidence-based infant nap guidelines'. Science simply does not know how long babies should sleep for in the daytime and how many naps they should have per day. At most, the best advice a parent can be given is to monitor their baby's sleep cues and tiredness signs and to be baby-led when it comes to daytime sleep. If babies are tired then ideally parents will help them to sleep. If they are not tired, it doesn't matter what a random table says: parents should not try to make them sleep. Following the individual needs of babies is a far better guide for daytime sleep than any opinion, expert or otherwise.

Research[10] does exist that shows the average amount of daytime sleep taken at differing ages. This research can provide a very rough guide for parents to know what to expect. It is, however, incredibly important to understand that these numbers do not indicate how much sleep babies should get. There are no 'shoulds' in this research: the scientists observed many babies to arrive at an average figure for the amount of time they spent napping at different ages. There will always be babies who need more naps than the average, just as there will always be babies who need fewer. A baby who does not

Age of Baby	Average Total Daytime Sleep
1 month	5 to 6 hours
3 months	4 to 5 hours
6 months	3 to 4 hours
9 months	2 to 3 hours
12 months	2 to 3 hours

fit into the 'averages' is most likely still having their daytime sleep needs met.

At each age there are no evidence-based guidelines for how many naps a baby should have. Similarly there are no evidence-based guidelines for the maximum number of hours a baby should be awake for *between* naps, although both of these greatly concern parents.

Once again the most important advice for parents is to be led by their baby. Some babies prefer several short naps, often only lasting for one sleep cycle. Others prefer a nap to last for two or three sleep cycles, and may take all of their daily sleep need in one or two longer naps. There is no right and wrong when it comes to naps. The most important figure to consider is the total sleep need of a baby in a twenty-four hour period. Babies who sleep for longer at night are likely to need less sleep in the day and vice versa.

The dreaded nap drop

As babies' circadian rhythms begin to mature, they will begin to consolidate their night-time sleep. Daytime naps will naturally lessen in both length and frequency as night-time sleep becomes longer, with fewer periods of waking, resulting in less of a need for daytime sleep.

As babies grow, the reduced need to take naps in the later afternoon has an important effect on night sleep. The rationale behind this is to build enough of a sleep drive, or need, so that the baby can fall asleep easily at night. If a large proportion of the baby's twenty-four hour sleep need is taken during the day then they will naturally need less sleep and wake more at night. The process of dropping naps is a representation of the baby's increasing neurological maturation. As the brain matures, the baby is able to tolerate more hours awake in the day. The dropping of a daytime nap is a good indicator that the baby's circadian rhythms are maturing and that their night-time sleep is beginning to look more like that of adults.

Despite this, however, many parents are keen for their baby to have more, or longer, daytime naps. These quiet hours alone in the day are often used for the parent to catch up on chores around the house, or sometimes to work. The dropping of a nap is commonly met with horror as parents mourn the loss of alone or adult time during the day, and many parents try to encourage their baby to sleep for longer than they need during the day. Baby sleep is not convenient! Babies do not nap to allow parents to have some time off, they nap because their brains need them to. As babies age their brains do not require as much daytime sleep. This is a simple fact of biology and one that really cannot be fought with any amount of artificial light blocking, driving cars, pushing buggies, lullabies or ignoring needs. If a baby is ready to drop a nap the best thing the parent can do is to accept it. On a related note, trying to schedule baby naps around daytime activities often doesn't end well. Daytime activities should be worked around baby naps, or parents may prefer to follow the lead of other cultures and continue their day with their sleeping baby held close to them in a sling or carrier, or use naps to take time out and rest with their baby. Just as these parents did:

'Our slings are the best baby purchase (we have three!), we all love them and use them for the same reason we bed-share. I just wish there were slings strong enough to carry my eight-year-old when we both need emotional refuelling.'

'I co-slept for some daytime naps so I could sleep too. Napping in a sling or on my chest was basically born out of necessity. The only other place he would sleep would be next to me in bed

which, lovely as that is, isn't practical when you need to actually do stuff.'

'I spent the first six months of my son's life so conflicted by all the advice I received on getting my baby to sleep during the day. Most involved leaving my son to cry. I just couldn't do it. It didn't feel right. For months he would only sleep on my chest. Everyone told me it was a bad habit. Now at nine months he is rocked or breastfed to sleep and loves sleeping in his cot. I miss him sleeping on me! I think the best advice I was given was to surrender. Surrender to what feels best for you and your baby. You and your baby will be happier because of it.'

'For daytime naps my daughter preferred to be in a carrier. This also made it much easier with another child, only two years older, who wanted to play with me in the day.'

'Even though my little girl is now nine months old I still lie down and rest, sometimes nap, with her when she is napping. I am so grateful for this time as it allows me to be fully able to enjoy her when she's up and about.'

'I let my son nap in the sling guilt free. I thought I needed to get my first in a routine and she would cry a lot before she fell to sleep. I feel sure she was either overtired or not yet tired as I was following the clock and not her. My son shows signs of tiredness and I pop him in the stretchy wrap sling. He generally nods off when he's ready. He's also a lot happier, and so are the rest of us.'

'In the day when she needed a feed or a nap I had to sit on the sofa or on the bed and I had to rest. I had to sit there and feed and hold her for around an hour. This meant I had to rest throughout the day at regular intervals. Although this wasn't *sleep it did mean I managed to get some rest during the day, which helped me to cope with the nights.'*

'My baby does not have a pram, we choose to use slings on a daily basis. They mean that we have our hands free to play with our toddler and to get jobs done around the house. I can't even imagine trying to put him down for a nap! It's natural instinct for him to want to be close to his caregivers.'

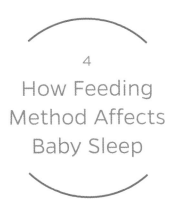

4

How Feeding Method Affects Baby Sleep

Do formula fed babies sleep better than breastfed babies? The age-old advice to '*give the baby a bottle to get them sleeping through*' has stood the test of time and is recommended by everybody from grandmothers to health professionals. But is there any truth in it? To answer the question we first need to understand the difference between breastfeeding and formula feeding when it comes to infant biology.

How breastfeeding affects sleep

Human babies are meant to drink human milk. This is not a judgement statement. I am not saying 'breastfeeding is best feeding'. This is a statement of fact. Breastfeeding is not 'best feeding', breastfeeding is 'normal feeding'. Human breastmilk is the only milk that is biologically appropriate to feed baby humans. Again there is no judgement intended in that statement. On a purely biological and evolutionary level it makes no sense to feed our babies milk from another species. Indeed, when we do feed our babies milk from cows or goats the milk has to go through quite complex processes in order to make it more suitable for human infant consumption. The result is a product that can be lifesaving if there are absolutely no other alternatives (donor milk from another lactating mother is a better alternative if breastfeeding from the baby's own mother is impossible), but it is vitally important that we do not think that infant formula is comparable to human breastmilk. It isn't.

Humans are by nature meant to be 'hunter gatherers'. Traditional societies still exist that can give us a good idea about how childcare was organised in the past, such as the nomadic Hadza of Tanzania. Commonly female gatherers would do so in a community of other women. Babies would be carried, either in arms or more likely with some form of cloth wrap. Alternatively babies would be held by other female members of the community, often younger sisters and nieces. Many mammals form community 'nurseries' of sorts where the babies are taken care of if the mother is away, particularly if the mothers of that species are hunters rather than gatherers. In these nurseries it is common for other lactating mothers to allow the temporarily motherless babies to feed from them. This occurs in many different species from seals to monkeys. The fact that human mothers gather is important, as despite the presence of community nurseries, most gatherers would have gathered with their babies with them. Gatherers do not tend to leave their babies for long periods of time, if at all. This evolutionary marker helps to define the consistency of our breastmilk. Human babies are meant to feed little and often. Our milk is easily digestible because our babies are not intended to be apart from us for long periods of time.

Contrast this to a seal and her pup. Seal milk is high in fat. Up to 60 per cent of the milk is composed of fat, a much higher percentage than in human milk, which contains between 3 and 5 per cent fat.[1] This ratio is indicative of the milk of a hunter. A hunter mother will at some point have to leave her baby for a long period of time without her milk, or in the hopes that another mother will allow the baby to feed from them. Similarly a hunter baby will wean from the mother at the earliest opportunity. In the case of a seal pup, weaning will occur at around six weeks of age. The fat content of human milk indicates that we are not meant to leave our babies for any length of time. Our babies should be fed often, during the day and night. Our young are also meant to nurse for longer. A gatherer baby will wean significantly later than a hunter baby.

Breastmilk is a living substance. As a baby's needs change, so the milk changes too. Breastmilk is full of antibodies and helpful bacteria to bolster the baby's immune system, which adapts as a result of the pathogens mother and baby are exposed to. Perhaps the most important difference between breastmilk and formula milk, however, is the way that the composition of breastmilk changes over the course of a day in response to the mother's circadian rhythm.

There are four important effects the mother's circadian rhythm has upon her milk. The first is the secretion of prolactin, the hormone primarily responsible for making milk. Prolactin secretion is significantly higher at night,[2] which means that breastmilk is produced in greater quantities at night. This explains why babies may feed more at night, as the milk is more plentiful. This is especially important for a baby who doesn't feed much in the day, perhaps due to the introduction of solids, a mother who has returned to work or because they are too distracted to feed much during the day. Secondly, night-time breastmilk contains melatonin,[3] the hormone of sleep. As the mother's melatonin levels rise in the evening, so do the levels in her breastmilk. This melatonin is then transferred to the baby during evening and night feeds and can help to 'top up' their immature circadian rhythm and increase melatonin levels, thus aiding sleep. Third, night-time breastmilk is also higher in tryptophan,[4] an amino acid which promotes the synthesis of serotonin. Serotonin in turn has a regulatory effect on circadian rhythms.

Circadian rhythm also affects night-time breastmilk through the presence of neuropeptides, small protein-like molecules, which act as chemical signals in the body and brain, including those related to sleep. There are three neuropeptides that are specifically related to sleep: 5'UMP, 5'AMP and 5'GMP. 5'UMP helps to increase the number of both REM and nREM episodes of sleep. 5'AMP works to induce sleep in the first place, and 5'GMP helps to regulate circadian rhythms. Research[5] has found that post-8pm breastmilk contains higher levels of 5'AMP, and the levels are particularly high in the hours up to midnight. Levels of 5'UMP are significantly higher in breastmilk in the middle of the night. Results also found fluctuating levels of 5'GMP in breastmilk over a twenty-four hour period. The raised levels of these three nucleotides at night indicates a further sleep inducing and circadian regulating effect of night-time breastmilk. It is important to note, however, that expressed breastmilk will only aid sleep if the milk is expressed at night.

How formula feeding affects sleep

Scientists have spent many years refining formula milk to be more suitable for human infants. At the beginning of the twentieth century, babies not fed breastmilk were often given mixes of cow's milk, sugar and water, a concoction clearly lacking in nutrients and inappropriate for babies. Recent advances have seen formula milk regularly improved in the pursuit of making it better meet the needs of babies. Some of these improvements include the manipulation of levels of long-chain polyunsaturated fatty acids, such as DHA, to levels more closely matched to those found in breastmilk and the fortification and improved bio-availability of important elements such as selenium.[6] However, formula milk is still incomparable to breastmilk, particularly in the way breastmilk adapts and changes to the baby's needs. There is no denying that it has come a long way from last century and no doubt will be further improved upon in the future.

When it comes to sleep, formula milk is significantly different to breastmilk. It does not contain melatonin. Nor does it contain tryptophan or the sleep-related nucleotides such as 5'AMP, 5'UMP and 5'GMP. There is no link between maternal circadian rhythm and formula feeding, no chemical cue that it is time to sleep. The formula milk babies are fed at night will contain exactly the same compounds as the milk they are fed in the morning. It may well be possible to engineer a 'night-time' formula milk to capitalise on some of the sleep-inducing qualities of breastmilk, and no doubt this idea is already being pursued by formula manufacturers. The lure of a 'sleep-inducing milk' and the extra profit that it would bring must be incredibly appealing. Research[7] already exists to show that it may be possible to fortify formula milk with some of the compounds that can affect sleep, particularly tryptophan and certain nucleotides. The research findings suggest that adding these components to formula milk improves baby sleep. The production of special 'night-time' formula would be another way to entice parents to spend money on baby milk and continue to line the pockets of the formula manufacturers and inventors.

Despite the lack of sleep-inducing compounds, there is one way in which formula milk can make a baby sleep more deeply and for longer. Formula milk is harder to digest than breastmilk. This is because the milk was originally intended for cows, rather than humans. (Most infant formulas are based on dried cows' milk powder.) This inter-species usage means that human babies find the milk harder to digest than calves, the intended recipient. While this difficulty in digesting may result in babies becoming sleepier, formula milk can also have the opposite effect. Some babies may be unsettled as their digestive systems work overtime, and constipation is more common in formula-fed babies, which can understandably cause discomfort and thus interrupted sleep. On a biological level, therefore, with all things considered, it doesn't make sense that formula-fed babies would sleep more than their breastfed counterparts.

What the research says

If popular opinion is to be believed, the quickest route to a full night's sleep is to feed formula milk rather than breastmilk, at least for the last feed of the day. Is there any truth in this widespread belief? It would seem not: the science tells a very different story. Research suggests that mothers who breastfeed, especially at night, get significantly more sleep than their formula-feeding counterparts. In addition, mothers who breastfeed seem to cope better with sleepless nights than those who formula feed.

Research[8] that looked at the sleeping patterns of mothers in the immediate postnatal period has found that breastfeeding mothers average thirty minutes more sleep at night than formula-feeding mothers by one month postpartum. Scientists have also found that exclusively breastfed two- to four-month-old babies had significantly less night-time colic and irritability than babies of the same age who were formula fed.[9] The breastfed babies slept significantly more than the formula-fed babies at night. These findings have been replicated many times, with researchers suggesting that much of this difference can be explained by the sleep-inducing chemical properties of breastmilk, which contains melatonin and tryptophan, as we have seen. This correlation was highlighted by a team of researchers[10] who not only found a greater level of sleep consolidation in breastfed babies, but also linked this sleep to increasing levels of tryptophan found in night-time breastmilk.

Breastfeeding is not only a marker of better infant sleep: researchers have also found a correlation with maternal sleep and maternal mood. One team of scientists[11] set out to measure cortisol levels during the day and night in breastfeeding and formula-feeding mothers. Their research found significantly less cortisol in the systems of breastfeeding mothers at night compared to those who were formula feeding, which they linked to the breastfeeding mothers' reports of lowered stress levels and fewer negative mood states than those who were formula-feeding. These findings confirm those of other research[12] which indicates lower levels of postnatal depression in breastfeeding mothers compared to those who formula feed. One of the reasons for this may be the ease with which breastfeeding mothers are able to feed at night: there is no need to fully awaken to prepare bottles, particularly if the baby is in, or next to, their own bed. Often night-time breastfeeding requires very little movement from the mother, which allows her to fall back to sleep again much more quickly than a formula-feeding mother. Thus, although night-time breastfeeds may be frequent, in most cases they are far less disruptive to the breastfeeding mother's sleep than formula feeds.

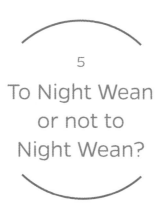

5

To Night Wean or not to Night Wean?

Does night weaning improve baby sleep? Many believe it does. Those who offer sleep advice based on behavioural theory suggest that parents should not 'reward the baby' by feeding them milk at night. They insinuate that the baby is waking because of the milk. This is a naive and narrow view. As we have already seen, it is normal for babies to wake many times in the night. Indeed, it is impossible for them to 'sleep through', as their multiple sleep cycles demand exactly the opposite. It is a biological fact that babies will wake many times every night, just as adults do. The real issue is whether or not the baby can begin a new sleep cycle without parental input.

Babies do not wake in the night because they want milk. They wake because they have finished a sleep cycle. At the end of the cycle, when they become more alert, they may feel hunger or thirst and cry for a feed. This is common in the early months when their stomachs are small and particularly when milk is their exclusive food source. As babies grow and begin to approach their first birthday, it becomes more likely that they can transition between sleep cycles without needing to feed out of pure hunger. The naivety of the assumption that babies wake because of night feeds lies in the fact that we *don't actually know* why babies sometimes need parental help to transition between sleep cycles.

Not all babies who cry for their parents will be hungry. In fact the percentage that are hungry is probably significantly lower than many think during the latter half of the baby's first year. The reality is that feeding is much more than simple nutrition for babies. Suckling is incredibly calming and can soothe even the most fractious of babies. Babies may use night feeds as a way to alleviate pain, such as that felt during teething. They may use night feeds as a way to reconnect with a mother who has been absent or busy during the day. Babies may use night feeds as a way to feel safe and secure, particularly during phases of separation anxiety and developmental leaps. None of these reasons are to do with hunger, yet the solution is the same: feeding. If you stop night feeding you do not take away these non-hunger-related needs. You are left with them, and the quickest and easiest way to resolve them has gone.

Night feeding is not a bad habit. Night feeding will not encourage a baby to wake more at night. Night feeding is not the cause of sleepless nights. Sleeping next to breasts does not encourage a baby to wake more. Babies sleeping like babies is the cause of sleepless nights; night feeding is just something that can help. Believing that stopping night feeds is 'the answer' to infant night waking illustrates the ignorance of those suggesting it. In the previous chapter we saw how breastfeeding can encourage night sleep, in both baby and mother. In many cases it is the *solution* to frequent night waking, not the cause.

What happens if babies are fed more in the day, particularly solids? Again, along with night weaning, this recommendation is commonplace. Parents are advised to 'fill up' their babies as much as possible during the day, with both milk feeds and solids. The assumption is that the more that the baby eats during the day, the fuller they will feel at night and the less likely they will be to wake. Parents are often advised to introduce solids into the baby's diet earlier than the normal and recommended six-month point. Again this advice stems from the belief that night waking is always due to hunger. Fill the babies up as much as possible and the assumption is that they will sleep all night. It is an incorrect assumption and shows very little understanding of infant needs and physiology.

Recent research[1] has attempted to investigate the link between night feeds, solids intake and infant wakings. Researchers studied the sleep patterns of over 700 babies aged between six and 12 months old. The mothers were asked to report their babies' night wakings and night feeds, in addition to providing details of daytime food intake, both milk and solids. The results revealed that almost 79 per cent of six- to twelve-month-old babies still woke regularly at night, and that 61 per cent of the babies still had at least one milk feed per night. There was no difference in night wakings and night feeds between babies who were breastfed and babies who were formula fed. The most interesting finding of the research, however, was that those babies who consumed more solid food and milk during the day didn't feed as much at night as those who consumed less in the day. At first glance this seems to support those who advise 'filling up during the day'. However, the research showed that while babies who fed lots in the day didn't feed as much at night, they did wake just as much as those who still had night feeds. In other words, *night feeds had no impact on night wakings.* So, contrary to popular opinion, we now know that night weaning does not improve night sleep. The research also busted another common myth, that formula-fed babies sleep better than those who are breastfed.

These findings have been echoed by further research,[2,3] which investigated the impact of introducing solids into a baby's diet on their sleep. Neither study found any difference in night waking between babies who had been weaned onto solids and were given them before bedtime, and those who were exclusively fed a milk diet or who had not received any solids in the run-up to bedtime. Babies wake because they are babies. Babies don't wake because they are fed at night. They are not motivated to wake regularly because of the promise of a breast or a bottle.

Do babies naturally night wean?

Some parents fear that if they do not night wean their baby, the baby will be feeding during the night forever more. Although it is true that babies naturally outgrow the need for night feeds, from both a physical and a psychological perspective, for new parents that day can seem a long way off. Towards the latter half of their first year babies may seem to be feeding in the night more than ever and parents start to lose hope. But if we think about the developmental changes that older babies are going through, the reasons for their frequent desire to feed are understandable. Perhaps the most important of these changes is the onset of separation anxiety.

Separation anxiety commonly starts to affect babies at around eight or nine months of age, and it can be a scary time for them. During this period, they realise that you can leave them, but they don't know when, or even if, you are coming back. The constant worry about being abandoned can cause them to need you more than they ever have. This deep emotional need is commonly met by something that has comforted them since the day they were born: milk feeds. As the baby develops emotionally other means of comfort can help, and the need for night feeds wanes naturally. The period between 12 and 24 months of age often sees a fairly dramatic decrease in night feeds, entirely of the baby's own accord, without any need for parentally instigated night weaning.

What if you want to night wean?

Although science shows us that babies do not sleep better after the introduction of solids or night weaning, many mothers decide that the time has come to reduce or stop night feeds, perhaps so that somebody else can help in the night or sometimes because they are simply feeling 'touched out' – overwhelmed by the physical demands of motherhood.

The decision to night wean is not one to be made lightly. The process can be stressful for all family members, and in some cases can make nights harder, not easier. There are no guarantees the baby will sleep better; sometimes their sleep regresses and parents are left without alternative ways to soothe the baby. Making an informed choice that has considered all the pros and cons is important. It is not a decision that should ever be made after a particularly bad night. There are four important questions you should ask yourself before you decide to night wean.

1. Why do you want to night wean?

If your answer here centres on the opinions or advice of others, be they friends, family or professionals, then you absolutely should not night wean. The only person who can decide when to night wean – aside from your baby – is you. Nobody else knows the intricacies of your family and the relationships within it. Most advice to night wean given to parents is opinion, not evidence-based and is factually incorrect. The decision must stem from your own desire, never that of somebody else.

2. Do you want to night wean because you are exhausted?

If the answer to this question is 'yes', this is not the right time for you to night wean. Night weaning may mean your baby needs you more and not less during the night. Without being able to offer a breast or bottle you are likely to find it much harder to get them back to sleep. You are likely to have to get up out of bed and you are likely to be much, much more tired. Night weaning is hard work, both emotionally and physically. A much better solution here would be to look elsewhere to help with your exhaustion first. Spend some time working on yourself and taking care of your needs. They are much easier to meet than your baby's will be without night feeds.

3. Do you want to night wean because you are returning to work?

This is a very common trigger for night weaning. Many parents rightly believe that they will be able to cope with their return to work more easily if they get more sleep at night. Many believe that this better sleep will happen as a result of night weaning. Research, however, disproves this point. Night weaning and returning to work may even cause the baby's sleep to regress, when they do something known as 'reverse cycling'. Reverse cycling describes the baby's need to reconnect with you, largely by feeding, after a period of separation. Allowing the baby to reconnect by staying close and feeding at night can help to soothe any disconnect they may have felt by being away from you during the day. In turn this will commonly reduce any regression that may occur in their sleep. Night weaning and returning to work can often result in a baby who wakes more than normal, and a parent who has no easy way to settle them. For mothers who are breastfeeding night feeds are a particularly important way to help ensure the continuation of breastfeeding when the mother returns to work.

4. Do you want to night wean because you want another baby?

Night feeds are commonly seen as a barrier to conceiving another baby. In many cases the decision to night wean rests on the desire to fall pregnant. There is no specific number of hours in a row that you should not breastfeed for if you want your fertility to return. This differs from woman to woman. Some will regain full fertility while exclusively breastfeeding both day and night, while others will not regain their full fertility until after all breastfeeding ceases. Shortening feeds (and suckling time), or stretching out feeds, may help in some cases, but in others pregnancy doesn't happen until the baby has weaned both in the night and day. Weaning does not have to happen specifically at night in order for pregnancy to happen. In many cases reducing feeds during the day while continuing to feed as normal during the night can see the return of fertility. This is a pattern that is often observed as babies approach toddlerhood, when they become too busy and pre-occupied to feed much during the day. The most important question to ask here is whether there is a reason to rush to conceive again, or if you can wait another six months or so. Six months is not much time in your life, but to your baby it is an eternity. Those six months can go a long way towards meeting their needs, while postponing yours for only a short while.

Ideally, parentally instigated night weaning will also

happen at a point when there is no other stress present for the baby. This means taking into account, and avoiding, the following periods:

- teething
- separation anxiety
- starting daycare
- after a period of illness
- immediately before or after going on holiday
- any big physical developments, such as learning to crawl

How to night wean

There are no universal ways to night wean that work for each family. Indeed the 'best' night weaning method is one that has been devised with your unique family in mind. Some families decide to night wean while sharing a bed with their baby, in order to provide constant physical reassurance when night feeds are removed. Others decide to night wean with the baby in their own sleeping environment in order to reduce the confusion that may occur when they are sleeping right next to the source of milk. Some families utilise daddy cuddles, to provide some reassurance in lieu of feeds while mum sleeps in a different room. Some families wean over a quick period, feeling that this minimises the stress that the baby will experience compared to spreading the weaning over a longer period. Others prefer to take a slow but sure approach, gradually reducing night feeds over several weeks or even months. The decision depends on many factors, including current sleeping arrangements, who is present in the family home and any time pressures looming.

What is important, however, is to always make sure that the baby is not left with nothing that comforts them. If you draw a pie chart of 'things that calm babies in the night', for most regular night feeders it would look like this:

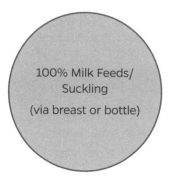

The aim with night weaning is to slowly reduce the percentage of soothing provided by night feeds, via the introduction of other ways to calm the baby. The pie chart then begins to resemble something like this:

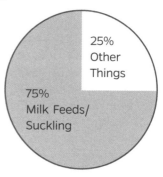

Before the actual process of reducing or spacing feeds at night happens, it is important to introduce the 'other things' before taking away the baby's sole source of comfort – night feeds. These 'other things' should be introduced for several weeks before night weaning in order that the baby can begin to take comfort from them before they need to rely on them alone. These 'other things' may include:

- A comfort object such as a blanket or cuddly toy.
- Some relaxing music or white noise.
- A scent, particularly one that they associate with the mother.
- A consistent and reassuring bedtime routine.
- Cuddles with dad.
- A special, sleep-friendly, bedtime light source.
- Reassuring words.
- A cup or bottle of water (in case of thirst).

The aim is that all of these 'other things' are easily accessible in the middle of the night at a time when the baby may ordinarily need a feed. It is even better if the baby can access them without parental involvement, which may mean that they can transition between sleep cycles without waking fully and crying. Initially the 'other things' may mean a very small reduction in night feeds, but as the baby derives more and more comfort from them the pie chart will slowly begin to change until ultimately 'other things' may reach up to 95 per cent of 'things that calm baby in the night'. Sometimes, however, the odd night feed will still be needed, especially if the baby is ill or very distressed for some reason, as it is likely they will remain the source of comfort most soothing to the baby for quite some time. Some parents may decide that they are happy if their pie chart goes from 100 to 50 per cent and that this shift will allow them to leave the decision to night wean fully to be completely baby led, which ultimately is always the best, and indeed easiest, way to night wean.

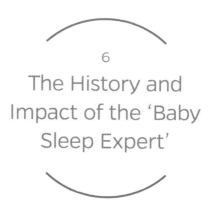

6

The History and Impact of the 'Baby Sleep Expert'

In life we have a tendency to trust professionals. We believe that their expert understanding is superior to ours. In many cases this is true. We would be wise to employ an electrician to rewire our home, and we would be wise to visit a dentist when we have a toothache. In either case carrying out the work ourselves could prove dangerous. These people have spent years training to learn their trade, they have passed externally regulated examinations, hold recognised qualifications and have appropriate insurance policies in place. Their practice is evidence-based and they continue to hone their skills and their knowledge through the years.

Parenting experts, however, are a whole new ball game. On the one hand we have medical doctors who believe they know all there is to know about raising children. Their medical degrees may afford them an understanding of paediatrics – the way a healthy child's body should function, and how to treat them when they are ill. What doctors don't have, however, is any in-depth knowledge of child psychology or day to day childcare. This is not an integral part of their training, and never has been. Doctors do not spend time during their medical training understanding normal sleep cycles, learning about the effects of different types of feeding or the ins and outs of bedsharing and the short and long term psychological effects of sleep training. While a plumber may have basic knowledge of electrical wiring, you wouldn't ask them to rewire your home. Yet this is precisely what many do when they take childcare advice from medical doctors. What many parents don't realise is that the childcare advice given by most health professionals is based entirely on their own opinions, which are often outdated or incorrect. Their professional status makes them dangerous, because it makes them trustworthy.

Then we have the self-proclaimed 'baby sleep expert'. There is no standard training or qualification for this role. There are no unbiased governing bodies overseeing practice. While organisations may exist that profess to regulate the work of sleep trainers, they are all developed and run by self-proclaimed 'sleep experts'. Anybody can set up a governing body. If I wanted to set up the 'International Association of Parenting Book Writers' I could do so tomorrow; there are no legal hoops to jump through and nobody to regulate me. I could design a logo and charge a fee for members to join my organisation. They could use my logo on their books, business stationery and websites to give their work an air of authority. Most people would not even think to check the validity and ethics of my association. This is the way that the baby sleep industry works. It is highly commercial and completely unregulated. Having read this book you could call yourself a 'baby sleep expert' and set up your own consultancy tomorrow. There would be nobody to stop you.

The baby sleep industry preys on the vulnerability of new parents. So many parents admit that they lost all touch with reason and logic in the sleep-deprived haze of parenting a newborn. I work with many psychologists who, when they become mothers themselves, admit to having consulted baby sleep trainers and followed their advice, despite having a huge amount of professional knowledge that runs contrary to what they are being advised. They describe the fear they have of not following the advice of 'the expert', even though it goes against their instincts and professional knowledge. They say they worry that if they don't do what 'the expert' advises, then they may create hideous sleep problems and an unhappy child. If these professionals, with in-depth knowledge of children and their needs, do not trust their instincts or education, then what hope do other parents have?

Baby sleep experts understand how desperate new parents are for two things: sleep, and a happy and healthy child. They promise to help parents to get their baby 'sleeping through the night' in a week or less. They tell parents that their advice is important so that their baby doesn't develop bad habits or miss out on learning the skill of 'being able to put themselves to sleep'. This mix of fear and promise sucks in even the least gullible. The parents, suffering from sleep deprivation and worrying about having sole responsibility for the life of this beautiful new baby, are easily duped and make very easy customers when it comes to 'the sell'.

These parents describe how they felt on the receiving end of advice from 'experts', whether from a book, or in person:

'I read a lot of 'parent-led' parenting books whilst pregnant. It was clear early on that it wouldn't work for my daughter, but I felt like a sap for not enforcing their methods. I was made to feel that my daughter's poor sleep was my own fault for 'making a rod for my own back'. It took a while to become confident that baby-led approaches are valid and that doing things the hard

way (for me), to give my daughter what she needed, did not make me a bad parent.'

'I remember sitting on the side of the bed crying when my baby wouldn't go to sleep on his own at three weeks old! I thought I had made a terrible mistake by rocking him to sleep.'

'In the early days I felt guilty for breastfeeding my baby to sleep. I had read in a book that I shouldn't do it as it created bad habits. I didn't tell people that I would let him fall asleep like that, but I still felt guilty about it, until I learnt more about the properties of breastmilk and how natural what we were doing actually was!'

'When my first baby was born I felt dreadful for resorting to co-sleeping because all the parenting books and magazines I had seen advised against it.'

'All of the books, blogs and sleep coaching websites made me feel terrible. I would spend ages bouncing and walking my baby to get him 'drowsy but awake' because that's what they told me to do. I was too scared to let him fall asleep in my arms.'

'Most articles and most books make you feel bad. In fact I would say 90 per cent of places you look for advice make you feel lousy about creating so called bad habits, it is very much the minority that doesn't.'

'I was told by an expert to never let my baby breastfeed to sleep. I was told he would associate sleeping with feeding and to feed him only when he woke up. I made myself feel guilty from actually listening to the advice when I needed to be actively listening to my child's cues.'

It is in the interests of 'the baby sleep expert' to promote the idea that babies can sleep better earlier than the research shows. It is important that parents perceive that their baby is 'a poor sleeper'. If parents believe they have a poor sleeper, they are more likely to use the services of the 'expert'. Educating parents about the reality of normal baby sleep does the 'experts' out of business. In order to be potential customers parents need to be told that they are creating bad habits or relying on sleep props or crutches that will cause all sorts of problems in the future. They need to be told that sleep is incredibly important to their child's health and that they are unlikely to be getting enough of it. Parents need to be told that 'self-soothing' is an important skill that their baby needs to be taught, and that if they don't teach their baby properly, they will never sleep through the night. Coupled with these dire consequences 'the expert' must also make parents believe that there is some sort of magic recipe for getting babies to sleep better. The parents must believe that the pursuit of better sleep is complicated, and best handled with expert guidance. The 'expert' must lead the parents to believe that they have all sorts of knowledge that the parent doesn't, and cannot hope to gain from other sources. The truth, however, is that there are no magic secrets that will make babies sleep 'better'. If there were, they wouldn't be secret for very long.

This manipulation of parental emotions is not new. 'Experts' have been making a living selling falsehoods and false hope for generations. While the nature of advice tends to be cyclical, shifting between an authoritarian, harsher style, and an authoritative, gentler style, it is ever present and ever profitable. For centuries parenting wisdom was shared among women. Grandmothers, aunts and older sisters and cousins would take new mothers under their wing. Villages would embrace their new mothers, not only supporting them physically, but also emotionally. These are the true parenting experts. Those who have been there and trodden the path before, often many times. Those who learned from their own mistakes, those who desire to help other mothers for no reason other than that they respect and love them. This maternal matrix, however, is almost extinct, thanks in part to the increasing role of external 'experts'.

The parent-centric years: 1890–1940
Dr Emmett Holt

Luther Emmett Holt, or Emmett as he was more commonly known, is credited with being one of the first parenting experts. Born in 1855 in New York, Holt had a traditional Puritan upbringing. He trained as an American medical doctor, specialising in paediatrics, and later went on to co-found the American Pediatric Society, standing as president of the organisation on two occasions. Holt was a dedicated doctor and passionate about the care of babies and children, but many of his theories now seem a little misguided. Holt's first book, *The Care and Feeding of Children*, published in 1894, remains his most renowned and best-selling work.

Holt advocated a rigid, parent-led feeding schedule, stating that babies should never be at the breast for more than twenty minutes at a time, feeds were to be spaced to three hourly as soon as possible, and night feeds should be completely stopped by five months of age. Holt believed that crying was good for babies and that newborns should be made to cry regularly throughout the day in order to expand and exercise their lungs. He believed that habitual attention-seeking crying from babies should be completely ignored by the parents.

Holt believed that babies who cried to be held or rocked, or those who cried outside of his prescribed feeding schedule, or who weren't ill, were being manipulative. He advised parents to ignore them, saying '*It should simply be allowed to 'cry it out.' This often requires an hour, and in extreme cases, two or three hours. A second struggle will seldom last more than ten or fifteen minutes, and a third will rarely be necessary*'. Holt also warned of dire consequences of sharing a bed with a baby: '*If the infant sleeps with the mother, there is always the temptation to frequent nursing at night, which is injurious to both mother and child*'. Despite the unscientific nature of his claims, it is not too hard to spot the prevalence of Holt's theories in the advice of many modern-day 'experts'. Indeed, although we may have moved on from calling babies 'it', many still recommend that parents let their infants 'cry it out'.

Truby King

Three years after the birth of Emmett Holt another man was born who was to become highly influential in the world of childcare. Sir Frederick Truby King, better known as Truby King, was born in New Zealand in 1958. Truby King was a surgeon and lecturer in mental health. He spent time in charge of a lunatic asylum, where he was widely praised for his mental healthcare reforms and consideration of the needs of his patients. This period led to an increasing interest in psychology, which saw King branch out into paediatrics and in particular the emotional health of babies.

In 1907 King founded the Plunkett Society, which aimed to improve the lives of babies by teaching the public about proper care and nutrition, largely via the appointment of specialist nurses known as 'Karritane Nurses'. The Plunkett Society is still very much in existence in New Zealand today, as are Karritane Nurses. King's most famous book, *Feeding and Care of Baby*, advocated a strict feeding schedule, with four-hourly feeds only. If babies cried in between feeds they were to be ignored, whether night or day. King advised parents to only hold their baby when they were feeding them or changing their nappy. At other times they weren't to be interfered with and should be left to sleep alone. King's theories were devoid of love and nurturing; indeed, he believed these to be bad habits that should be avoided.

The child-centric years: 1940–mid 1980s

John Bowlby

Edward John Mostyn Bowlby, better known as John Bowlby, was a British psychoanalyst and psychiatrist who lived from 1907 to 1990. Bowlby is commonly referred to as the founding father of 'Attachment Theory', largely due to his work during the Second World War, in which he focussed on the importance of attachment between child and parent, which he believed to be hard-wired in the baby from birth. Bowlby believed that the roots of adult mental health lay in childhood, and for this reason considered the early years of extreme importance. Bowlby's work highlighted the trauma felt by babies when separated from their parents, particularly the mother.

Bowlby highlighted the baby's innate need to form a close bond with their mother and how the baby viewed her as a 'secure base' from which to explore the world. Bowlby's theories completely overturned the popular parent-centric thinking of the previous fifty years and brought about a new, child-centric way of parenting.

Donald Winnicott

From the 1940s to the 1960s British paediatrician Donald Winnicott made regular broadcasts on the topic of motherhood and parenting for the BBC. It was during these broadcasts that Winnicott focussed on the term the 'good enough mother'. Winnicott's concept of the good enough mother allowed mothers to lessen any guilt they felt about parenting. Rather than aiming to be perfect, Winnicott said, mothers should aim to be 'good enough', implying that their small 'failings' to meet their baby's needs actually allowed the baby to grow and become independent.

Winnicott encouraged mothers to trust their instincts when it came to raising their children, and focussed on the importance of nurturing and love. Winnicott's training in psychoanalysis led him to carefully consider the impact of the mother's feelings upon the baby, and of the baby's upon the mother. He knew that emotional health was just as important as physical health and encouraged mothers to be mindful of both.

Dr Benjamin Spock

Doctor Benjamin Spock (1903–98) was an American paediatrician famed for his more gentle approach to childcare. Spock encouraged affection and trusting parental instincts, and is famous for telling mothers to trust themselves, saying 'You know more than you think you do'. Spock's advice continued Winnicott's theme of the empowerment of mothers.

Spock's book, the *Common Sense Book of Baby and Child Care*, published in 1946, quickly become known worldwide and still topped the bestseller lists many years after publication, having sold over fifty million copies to date. The book encouraged parents to forget strict routines and to become more flexible and focus on the needs of their children.

Dr Penelope Leach

Born in 1937, the British psychologist Penelope Leach continued the child-centric theme of parenting in her book *Your Baby and Child: From Birth to Age Five*, published in 1977.

Leach encouraged parents to be baby-led and to listen to their instincts, rather than establishing a strict parent-led routine. She is famous for saying '*Whatever you are doing, however you are coping, if you listen to your child and to your own feelings, there will be something you can actually do to put things right or make the best of those that are wrong*.' Leach is quick to encourage parents to comfort their babies and is an outspoken critic of 'cry it out'.

The parent-centric years again: mid-1980s–present day
Dr Richard Ferber

Famous for introducing the world to 'cry it out', sometimes known as 'Ferberisation', Dr Richard Ferber is an American paediatrician who manages a large hospital paediatric sleep unit. Ferber's infamous book *Solve Your Child's Sleep Problems* was published in 1985 and remains a perennial bestseller.

Gina Ford

In 1999 British maternity nurse Gina Ford published *The Contented Little Baby Book*. Ford's book is in many ways reminiscent of the earlier teachings of Holt and King, with a strict parent-led schedule imposed upon the baby from only two weeks of age. Ford's complicated schedules change frequently based upon the baby's age. She is keen to point out that babies should not be allowed to form bad sleep associations that may inhibit their sleep, and for this reason discourages common night-time parenting techniques such as feeding to sleep. Ford believes babies are capable of 'sleeping through' the night from very early on and this is encouraged in her writings, occasionally through a process of controlled crying.

Tracy Hogg

Tracy Hogg was another British maternity nurse who died

in 2004. Hogg's legacy remains in her bestselling book *The Secrets of the Baby Whisperer*, which was published in 2001. The *Baby Whisperer* book is commonly described as a 'gentler alternative to Gina Ford', and at first look this seems accurate. Further reading, however, reveals that this is another parent-centric, routine-led book, which encourages independent 'sleeping through the night' as soon as possible. Hogg's method of sleep training centres on 'pick up, put down', a method that aims to train babies to eventually stop crying and go to sleep without parental input by constantly putting them down awake in their cot and only briefly picking them up to soothe them when they cry. Like Ford's techniques, the Baby Whisperer book has been frequently criticised for its incompatibility with successful breastfeeding.

One way of trying to understand the changes in parenting trends is to investigate how they reflect changes in society. The change to a more child-centric way of parenting can also be linked to the introduction of automatic washing machines, electric ovens, vacuum cleaners and other household appliances. These time-saving devices may have meant that mothers had more time to spend with their children, which may go some way towards explaining the more gentle approach prevalent from the 1940s until the mid to late 1980s. The late 1980s saw more and more mothers returning to the workplace, in many cases as a direct response to the precarious economic situation at the time and the need for higher household incomes. The increasing number of working mothers and children in childcare has meant that babies must fit into parents' routines and not vice versa. Mothers need their babies to sleep well so that they can get enough sleep at night, in order to work the next day. Our busy lives leave little time for meeting the needs of young babies.

Perhaps the next shift in parenting trend will not occur until parenting is shared more equally between men and women, our governments support stay at home mothers properly, or technology allows mothers to work from home in roles that offer flexi-time.

Is the next child-centric era due? Previous trends have tended to shift every forty years or so; perhaps the 2020s will bring a paradigm shift to a more gentle and compassionate style of parenting, particularly when it comes to coping with baby sleep. Importantly, perhaps for the first time, this shift will be backed by a vast amount of scientific research. Is this the key to making a child-centric approach 'stick' for the long-term?

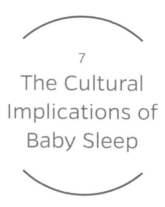

7

The Cultural Implications of Baby Sleep

There is no doubt that the society we live in impacts on our expectations and experience of baby sleep. Baby sleep problems do not appear to be universal; parents in Western countries seem to struggle the most. The key question to ask is whether babies in other cultures sleep differently, or are the differences in experience due to parental behaviour or expectations? To answer this question it is important to understand the differences in approaches to infant sleep around the world. What do parents in other countries do? Are other cultures set up to be more supportive of young families? Are other cultures more accepting of normal infant sleep? Do babies sleep at different times, or in different locations, depending on where they live? This chapter aims to investigate all of these questions and to discover if we can learn from other cultures and find ways to improve baby sleep and our handling of it.

Expectations of baby sleep around the world

Although there are often striking differences in the expectations of infant sleep among different cultures, one universal truth remains: all new parents struggle with their baby's sleep at some point. While expectations may differ between countries and cultures, babies still sleep like babies. Although all parents struggle with sleepless nights, the struggle does appear to be worst among predominantly Caucasian parents. Do Caucasian babies sleep differently? Or does the cause of the struggle perhaps lie with the expectations of the parents?

I don't think it is a coincidence that 'baby sleep experts' are predominantly Caucasian. All of the worldwide best-selling baby sleep books are written by white Americans, Australians or Europeans. The easiest way to write a best-selling sleep book is to promise an easy, quick fix for baby sleep. Words such as 'secret', 'miracle' or 'solution' are prominent in titles and book blurbs. The unregulated, self-styled 'baby sleep trainers' are almost entirely Caucasian too. In order to sell sleep books or services it is first necessary to define a problem. If there is no problem then there is no need or demand for the books or services. If there is no problem there is no monetary gain to be made and there are therefore no career options in the field.

Along with the experts, authors and trainers, Western society profits hugely from unrealistic expectations of baby sleep. If parents understood that their baby did not have a sleep problem then they would not seek out the latest gadgets to try to 'fix' them. Special sleep-inducing story books, sleep training clocks, hammocks, noise machines, rockers, light shows, glowing animals, sleeping bags and swaddles promising better sleep would have no market. It is in the interests of the economy that sleep is sold as a problem needing to be fixed. The issue is that the demand is based upon a need that doesn't actually exist. The sad truth is that it is not economically viable to re-educate Western parents on infant sleep.

Many countries consider night feeding normal long beyond

the current Western norm. There is no rush to night wean, no quest to teach 'self-soothing'. It is accepted that human infants need to feed at night and will wake often to do so. This need is met without question, just as the baby's need for parental proximity at night is not debated. Many societies understand that it is normal for babies to wake regularly at night and therefore parents seek not to change the baby's sleep, but to alter their own behaviour. In many cultures parenting is an extended family activity. Motherhood is rightly valued and mothers are supported to care for the normal needs of their babies. In many ways our quest for 'equal opportunities' in the workplace in our society has devalued the role of motherhood. Many mothers return to work shortly after birth and struggle to meet the demands of their job and the demands of their baby. Balancing childcare and a busy household is hard work. Something has to give. All too often, sadly, it is the needs of the baby. The baby who is sleeping 'like a baby', but whose busy working parents need him to sleep like an adult.

Where babies sleep around the world

In Korea, research[1] has found that 88 per cent of infants will share a sleep surface with their parents. Co-sleeping in Korea is common and seen as culturally acceptable and an important part of parenting. In Japan[2] over two-thirds of babies share a sleep surface with their parents. The same research indicates that only 15 per cent of American babies do the same. In Egypt[3] almost 70 per cent of infants sleep with their parents and research has shown that these babies wake less during the night than their solitary sleeping counterparts. In New Zealand just under 6 per cent of babies were found to sleep with their parents, whereas almost 84 per cent do in Vietnam. Further research,[6] which looked at the infant sleeping practices of 186 non-industrialised societies, found that 46 per cent of infants slept in the same bed as their parents, while a further 21 per cent slept in a separate bed, but still in the same room as their parents. In total 67 per cent of families in the non-industrialised societies studied slept with the children and parents in close proximity to each other.

In a study of 136 different societies, anthropologist John Whiting[7] reported an association he had discovered between the climate and co-sleeping. Whiting found that in countries with mild winters more parents sleep with their babies. In countries with cold winters babies were more likely to sleep alone. Presumably this is to enable wrapping of the babies and extra bedding for the parents. Of all the different permutations of co-sleeping, including mother sleeping with the child and the father elsewhere, and mother and father sleeping together with the child, Whiting found that the most common arrangement across all cultures, shared by approximately 50 per cent of all families studied, was that of the mother and child sleeping together and the father sleeping elsewhere. This is in stark contrast to the most common sleeping arrangement in our own society, where the mother and father sleep together and the baby sleeps elsewhere.

Mayan culture is well known for co-sleeping practices. Research by anthropologist Gilda Morelli[8] studied the sleeping habits of Mayan Indians living in Guatemala and compared them to those of Americans. She found that Mayan mothers all sleep with their babies until some point between their first and second birthday. Fathers tend to join the mother and baby in bed, or sometimes sleep in another bed with the family's older children. None of their American counterparts slept with their parents with any regularity, and by the time they reached three months old almost 60 per cent were already sleeping alone in their own room. The American mothers frequently reported tiredness due to having to be awake to feed their babies at night, while the Mayan mothers had no complaints about night feeds, since they breastfed while asleep in most cases. When the Mayan mothers were told about the American infants in the same research they showed alarm, dismay, pity and sadness at the idea of the infants sleeping alone. One was recorded as saying 'but there's someone else with them there, isn't there?' She simply could not believe that American mothers would put their babies to sleep in their own room alone. The Mayan mothers viewed co-sleeping with their infants as part of an important commitment they had made to their families and to their relationship with their children, and did not view it as a chore.

In Western, predominantly Caucasian, culture we tend to view bedsharing and co-sleeping in two extreme ways. The first is the idea that it is something that is outdated or unnecessary due to the invention of cots, which are viewed as an improvement and advancement on historical human sleeping practices. Comments such as 'We're not cavemen any more, why would we parent in such a way? It's time to move on and catch up with the times', are not uncommon. Other people consider sleeping with babies modern, 'new-fangled' and trendy. Mainstream media sources frequently run stories on the new 'co-sleeping fad', portraying it as a modern-day lifestyle choice, or a badge of honour for a certain style of parenting. The simple fact remains, however, that co-sleeping with our young is the biological norm for our species and indeed all mammals. Our tendency to have our babies sleep separately from us, either in their own container or own room, is at odds with our biology and evolution. There is nothing new or faddy about parenting the way nature intended. If there are any new fads or trends they are cots, cribs and Moses baskets. None of these are necessary for raising a human infant.

The timing of sleep around the world

If you travel the world and observe the bedtimes of babies in other cultures you are likely to see a very different pattern to that in Western societies. In the UK, the USA, Canada, Australia, New Zealand and other predominantly Caucasian societies acceptable bedtimes for infants tend to be around 6:30 to 7:30pm. It is common for parents to want to have the evening to themselves. This is adult-only time to recuperate from the day, rest from work, prepare meals, catch up on the internet or television programmes, clean and tidy, prepare for the next day and enjoy adult conversation. The Western desire to put children to bed early is a strong one. Are these early bedtimes in line with the needs of babies, however? What happens when parents persist in putting their baby to bed early, because of their desire to have an evening alone?

In most non-Caucasian countries bedtime for babies is significantly later. Research[3] has shown an average Egyptian bedtime occurring after midnight. In Hong Kong bedtime occurs on average at 10.15pm.[4] Asian countries in particular tend to have later bedtimes. Although bedtime for babies may begin much later than it does in the West, Asian mothers report that they sleep better and for longer than their Western counterparts.[5] In countries with later bedtimes babies spend their evenings with their parents, enjoying social activities, feeding and winding down 'in arms'. They tend to go to bed at the same time as parents, who do not prioritise evening time alone in the same way as those in Caucasian countries.

Are there any downsides to Western early bedtimes? If the baby is not tired it will simply be hard to get them to sleep. Settling will take longer and invariably be harder on the parent than if the baby was ready to sleep. Babies will commonly wake several times in the early part of the evening and perhaps need resettling every sleep cycle if they are not yet ready to sleep for the night. In many ways the quest for an early bedtime is harder on parents, as often they need to devote a significant proportion of their evening to getting the child to sleep and resettling them in the night. Similarly, if babies have fulfilled their sleep need they will wake, often very early, in the morning, which once again is at odds with parents' wishes. Not only do many parents wish for adult-only evenings, they also want their baby to sleep later in the mornings.

Research[9] has indicated that young children are biologically ready to sleep from roughly quarter past eight in the evening, with average sleep onset time occurring roughly half an hour later at a quarter to nine at night. This is the time that melatonin levels tend to rise to a level appropriate for sleep to begin. These findings certainly chime with the later bedtimes in other cultures, and seem very at odds with Caucasian expectations of the timing of bedtime, which are considerably out of sync with the circadian rhythms of children.

What would happen if Western families adopted the sleeping practices of other cultures? Would our 'sleep problems' be resolved by selecting a bedtime more in sync with our babies' circadian rhythms? Would our 'sleep problems' be resolved by allowing our babies to sleep in close proximity to us at night? Would parents feel less stressed and exhausted if they *accepted* their babies' needs, rather than fighting them in their quest to create independent, 'self-soothing', solitary sleeping babies? Or introducing night weaning prematurely? Once again we reach a point where we must question the validity of modern Western society's expectations when it comes to infant sleep. It seems that the problems that many experience with baby sleep are actually nothing to do with the baby, but everything to do with the warped and unrealistic way many believe, often through no fault of their own, their baby should sleep.

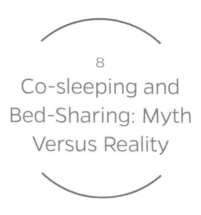

8
Co-sleeping and Bed-Sharing: Myth Versus Reality

If there is one element of night-time parenting that is shrouded in myth and mystery it is surely co-sleeping. Barely a month passes without a mainstream media source dredging up a 'Sharing a bed with your baby kills babies and marriages' story. Parent-centric baby experts pour scorn on the idea of a 'family bed' and warn of dire consequences of allowing your baby to sleep next to you. Messages from health professionals are also frequently muddled. Some categorically tell parents to never allow their baby into their bed, while others quietly encourage it in hushed tones, accompanied by backhanded advisory leaflets that they are not really 'meant' to distribute.

Co-sleeping versus bed-sharing

The terms co-sleeping and bed-sharing are often used interchangeably by parents, but they are quite different. For a proper discussion, particularly in terms of safety, it is vitally important that the terms are used correctly. To *co-sleep* with a baby means to sleep in the same room as them, but not necessarily on the same sleep surface. Co-sleeping can therefore include the baby sleeping in a Moses basket, crib or cot in the parents' bedroom, with the parents sleeping in their bed. Sometimes the baby's cot may be attached, or 'side-carred' to the side of the parents' bed. Co-sleeping also covers scenarios in which adults may have accidentally fallen asleep with their baby, such as in a nursing chair during a night feed, or on the sofa during a daytime nap when the parent has accidentally fallen asleep as well as the baby. The term *bed-sharing* is used solely to specify a parent sharing a bed with their baby.

Unplanned versus planned

It is important to further clarify the terms co-sleeping and bed-sharing with the sub-dividers 'planned' and 'unplanned'. Planned co-sleeping indicates a sleep environment where the parent has specifically chosen a night-time container for their baby close to their own bed and placed them to sleep in there. Planned bed-sharing describes a scenario in which the parent has researched bed-sharing and specifically arranged their bed and surrounding area in order to be as safe as possible for the baby. As we will discuss later in this chapter, both planned co-sleeping and planned bed-sharing are almost always *safe* for the baby and *beneficial* for parent and baby. Unplanned co-sleeping and unplanned bed-sharing, however, can be incredibly dangerous and should be avoided at all costs. In many cases carefully planning to co-sleep or bed-share will remove the risk of falling asleep in an unsafe manner with a baby accidentally. For instance, if parents are well rested they are less likely to accidentally fall asleep with their baby on the sofa or while feeding in a chair.

For the rest of this chapter we will specifically focus on the less well understood of the two practices: bed-sharing.

How many parents bed-share?

Incidences of bed-sharing are high throughout the world. Most parents will share a bed with their baby at some point during their parenting journey. In some countries bed-sharing is seen as the norm, while in others it is deemed unusual, or odd.

In the UK research estimates that at least half of all parents will share a bed with their baby at some point.[1,2] Research looking at Canadian[3] and American[4] sleeping arrangements put this figure closer to three-quarters of all families. Interestingly, the research has found that while very few parents anticipate sleeping with their baby before the birth, significantly more end up sharing a bed with their baby after the baby is born. This is a common trend that is of utmost importance for health professionals to understand, particularly when discussing the baby's sleeping environment with expectant or new parents. While most parents may feel strongly that bed-sharing is not for them while pregnant or when their baby is very newly born, it is highly likely that they will end up sharing a bed with their baby at some point during their first six months of life. For this reason it is vitally important that all parents, no matter what their initial plans, are taught how to bed-share safely.

Research shows that regular bed-sharing, where the baby's everyday place of sleep is in the parent's bed, is less common than occasional bed-sharing. While many parents may sleep with their baby during times when the baby is especially hard to settle, fewer choose to share their bed with their baby every night. Research[5] found that around a third of babies in Hong Kong regularly share their parents' bed. This is interesting when we consider the very low SIDS rate in Hong Kong of just 0.3 in every 1,000 live births, a rate significantly lower than that of the UK or the USA. This research echoes that from Japan,[6] which also highlights the normality of bed-sharing every night among families. In a comparison of the sleeping environments of American and Japanese children, researchers found that 59 per cent of Japanese children aged between six months and four years slept in their parents' bed at least three times per week. Further research[7] highlights the stark difference in bed-sharing rates between families in the East and those in the Western hemisphere.

While rates of regular bed-sharing remain low in predominantly Caucasian countries, research[8] indicates that the trend to bed-share is a growing one, despite frequent public health messages advising otherwise. This is a critical point for public healthcare policy makers to understand. Despite official guidance and highly emotive advertisements designed to dissuade parents from sharing a bed with their baby, rates are still rising. Research[9] has also indicated that only half of mothers share the details of their sleeping arrangements with their healthcare provider, meaning that many bed-share 'in secret'. It is high time those policy-makers understood that the way to protect lives is to educate parents so that they are supported to make informed choices as safely as possible. Especially if that choice is to bed-share.

Bed-sharing and breastfeeding – the perfect partnership

Anthropologists Professor James McKenna and Assistant Professor Lee Gettler believe so strongly in the synchronicity between breastfeeding and bed-sharing that they have coined a new term: 'breastsleeping'.[10] They use the term breastsleeping to describe the unique interplay between breastfeeding and infant co-sleeping. They believe strongly that bed-sharing should only be assessed in terms of safety when considered in combination with breastfeeding, as these two practices are the norm for our species. They feel that any measurement of infant sleep should use breastsleeping as the baseline from which to measure. In the absence of any known risk factors, breastsleeping is considered to be the most advantageous way to parent at night, for both baby and mother. They also rightly feel that healthcare professionals' attempts to prevent parents from sharing a bed with their baby, in the absence of known risk factors, are damaging to the breastfeeding relationship and thus the long-term health of mother and baby.

Why are breastfeeding and bed-sharing so closely linked? First, it is important to reiterate that these two behaviours are the norm for all mammals, including humans. We are meant to breastfeed and we are meant to sleep in close proximity to our infants. Anything else is deviating from the human biological norm and involves exposing our offspring to an element of risk. Breastfeeding alone significantly reduces the risk of Sudden Infant Death Syndrome (SIDS) by half at one month of age[11] when compared to formula feeding, so anything that can support breastfeeding can have a positive impact on the risk of SIDS.

Research[12] has found that mothers who bed-shared with their babies during the newborn period were twice as likely to still be breastfeeding when their baby was four months old as those who did not bed-share. These findings have been consistently echoed in those of other research,[13] where the relationship between bed-sharing and breastfeeding has been shown to last well into the child's second year of life.[14] This has led scientists to recommend that any discussions with parents about the risks of bed-sharing need to take into account the important relationship it has with breastfeeding and the impact this in itself has upon the risk of SIDS. From the mother's perspective, bed-sharing and breastfeeding are often the best and easiest ways to rest and sleep. The simple fact that very little effort is exerted by the mother – in terms of getting up to tend to the baby or prepare feeds – helps to consolidate the amount of sleep she gets at night and can go a long way towards boosting morale and energy levels. In addition, mothers who breastfeed tend to naturally sleep facing their baby, with the baby's head at breast height. This is widely recognised as the safest position for bed-sharing.

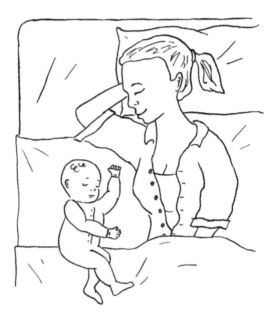

Is bed-sharing safe?

Unfortunately, there is no simple answer to this question. This explains why many large public health organisations, believing it important to disseminate one uniform, easy-to-understand message to all parents, dissuade parents from bed-sharing. It is true that in many instances bed-sharing can be extremely hazardous, but in the absence of known risk factors, research has shown no increased risk of bed-sharing compared to cot-sleeping. The difficulty lies in the fact that there is no single, definitive piece of research that proves bed-sharing to be safe or hazardous, which would reassure many professionals. The Academy of Breastfeeding Medicine is a global organisation of doctors who are dedicated to promoting, protecting and supporting breastfeeding. Their clinical protocol on co-sleeping and breastfeeding[15] states: '*There is currently not enough evidence to support routine recommendations against co-sleeping. Parents should be educated about risks and benefits of co-sleeping and unsafe co-sleeping practices and should be allowed to make their own informed decision.*'

Research[16] comparing a large number of cases of SIDS with a control group found that significantly more of the babies who had suffered from SIDS were co-sleeping than the babies in the control group. At first glance this research may appear to support the simple message that 'co-sleeping is dangerous'. However, when the results were studied in relation to specific co-sleeping environments, they painted a very different picture. The researchers found that certain co-sleeping practices, such as falling asleep with an infant on a sofa, having the baby in bed with a smoker, or with a parent who had consumed more than two units of alcohol, presented a very high risk to the baby. In the absence of these risk factors, however, there was no increased risk of SIDS. Based on these findings the authors argue that public health strategy should not try to dissuade all parents from sharing a bed with their baby, but should focus on making them aware of specific hazards and risks to avoid. UNICEF[17] corroborates this position, stating that: '*The issue of what to discuss with parents regarding parent-infant bed-sharing is controversial and confusing. Bed-sharing has advantages and dangers and views are informed by culture and personal belief. Simplistic messages in relation to where a baby sleeps should be avoided; neither blanket prohibitions nor blanket permissions reflect the current research evidence.'*

Common concerns about the safety of bed-sharing with babies include the issues of overheating, suffocation and overlaying. Several scientists are working to allay these fears. Research[18] studying the temperature of bed-sharing babies found that while they do tend to experience warmer external thermal conditions than their cot-sleeping contemporaries, they seem to be able to maintain a normal core body temperature. When it comes to suffocation, research[19] has found that the majority of bed-sharing babies studied spent at least a proportion of the night with their mouth and nose covered, in comparison to babies sleeping alone in cots, where the majority did not experience any airway covering. Despite this, however, researchers found there were no consistent effects on the babies' oxygen saturations or heart rate. Very similar findings were revealed in the same research when considering overlaying by a parent. In a third of all cases of bed-sharing parents rested limbs across their babies to some degree, but in cases where the full weight of the parent's limb was on the baby they moved and the parent removed the limb within fifteen seconds, thus presenting no danger to the baby.

The problems with current research

Bed-sharing research is fraught with difficulties and confusion. Research doesn't measure the same things, definitions tend to vary wildly and variables are missed, glossed over or data extrapolated. The majority of bed-sharing research is 'bad science' indeed. This leaves us in our current, unenviable position of having to critique each paper and try to piece together some semblance of understanding of the true position from a mismatched jigsaw puzzle.

Definitions present the first hurdle in bed-sharing research. Many researchers seem not to understand the difference between bed-sharing and co-sleeping, so research often does not differentiate between the two. The result is that sofa sleeping, which is highly dangerous, can be lumped in with bed-sharing. Amalgamated statistics therefore appear to show that all co-sleeping is dangerous, with the exception of the baby sleeping on their own in a cot in the parents' room. Sometimes researchers even consider an infant death to be caused by co-sleeping if the baby had previously bed-shared but actually died in their cot, which is frankly ridiculous. This confusion has led to the generation of incorrect blanket statements, used frequently in public health, including '*the safest place for a baby to sleep is in their own cot in the same room as the parents*'. Unfortunately the data does not exist to properly prove or disprove that statement, and it is misleading to pretend that it does.

The second stumbling block for co-sleeping research is that many researchers fail to determine whether the co-sleeping was planned or unplanned. Carefully planned bed-sharing is not in the same risk category as unplanned bed-sharing, hastily carried out with no thought at two in the morning with an exhausted parent who may not be thinking clearly. Yet in most research these two sets of circumstances are considered one and the same. Differentiate between planned and unplanned bed-sharing and the statistics will likely paint a very different picture. Furthermore, many studies do not record which parent the baby was sleeping with. Treating babies sleeping with fathers in the same way as babies sleeping with mothers overlooks the very different physiology of the two arrangements. The research also does not consider the positioning of the baby in the bed, and whether one or both parents were present. Having the baby in the middle of the bed presents an increased risk.

Most bed-sharing research does not determine whether mothers were breastfeeding, and thus whether babies may have been placed at more risk because of being formula fed. While most research pays lip service to variables such as alcohol consumption, smoking and medication usage, often not enough detail is recorded. For instance, the research does not think to ask whether the mother's *partner* had consumed alcohol or smoked, focusing instead almost solely on the mother. In the case of medication, questions often only focus on illegal recreational drugs, not prescription medication. This is a glaring omission, particularly with mothers of newborns, who are likely to be taking some form of post-birth analgesia.

Were mothers with long hair wearing their hair tied back? Were any ties on nightclothes kept well out of the way or removed? These questions all go unanswered in most of the research. Lastly, the sleeping environment itself is given little attention. The type of mattress and bedding used and location of the bedding and pillows in relation to the baby is not discussed. Unless research carefully considers all of these variables, it is impossible to come to any conclusions about the hazards posed by bed-sharing. Researchers who try to extrapolate public health messages from flawed research are naive at best and deceiving at worst.

Which risk factors should parents consider?

Our current understanding of bed-sharing research highlights the following risk factors that parents should make themselves aware of when planning to share a bed with their baby:

1. The mother should be breastfeeding. If the baby is formula fed they should have their own sleep surface.

2. Both parents should be non-smokers and the mother should not have smoked during her pregnancy.

3. Neither parent should have consumed alcohol in the 24 hours leading up to the bed-sharing.

4. Neither parent should have consumed recreational or prescription drugs, including post-natal analgesics, which may make them drowsy.

5. Neither parent should consider themselves to be 'excessively tired'. Some experts define this as fewer than five hours' sleep in the last 24 hours, while others feel this should be left to the parent to decide based upon their own instinct.

6. The mother should always sleep between her partner (and any older siblings) and the baby. The baby should never be placed in the middle of the bed between two adults.

7. Parents should always ensure that the sleeping surface is firm. Never fall asleep with a baby on a sofa, bean bag or water-bed. Memory foam mattresses should be avoided for the same reason.

8. The baby should be prevented from rolling off the bed. If possible parents should sleep on a mattress on the floor, or a futon-style bed low to the ground.

9. All pillows should be kept well away from the baby. The baby should always sleep at the same level as the mother's breasts, not her head.

10. The mother should lie on her side and form a protective frame around the baby with her body.

11. Duvets and blankets should be kept well away from

the baby to prevent the risk of smothering. Many mothers sleep in onesies or dressing-gowns to keep themselves warm.

12. Parents should ensure that the baby does not overheat; they should be dressed in appropriate clothing.

13. Parents with long hair should securely tie it back and should also not wear any nightclothes with loose ties or belts.

14. Parents should consider a separate sleeping surface if the baby is small for their age or is premature.

15. Parents should consider a separate sleeping surface if the mother is significantly overweight.

The benefits of bed-sharing

The benefits of bed-sharing are numerous. Most parents will cite 'more sleep', 'less stress' and 'easier feeding' as their primary reasons for bed-sharing. Many will say it was the only way the family could get a decent amount of sleep and most will say that they love snuggling with their baby at night. While it is true that babies who bed-share tend to wake more than those who are solitary sleepers, overall mothers who bed-share tend to get more and better quality sleep, especially as time spent awake, feeding and settling the baby is usually significantly shorter. Research[20] has found that overall bed-sharing mothers get an average of 8.6 hours' sleep per night, compared to their non-bed-sharing contemporaries who get 8.2 hours. The same research highlighted another benefit of bed-sharing: the babies experienced increased maternal touching and looking, increased breastfeeding, and faster and more frequent maternal responses in comparison to their non-bed-sharing counterparts. This increased nurturance is likely why many mothers report that their babies seem happier and calmer when sharing a bed with them. Research[21] has found that it isn't just mothers who are more nurturing when bed-sharing, however. Fathers also experience physical changes in their bodies in close proximity to their babies, which may help them to exhibit more nurturing behaviours. Scientists have found that fathers who bed-share experience a lowering of the hormone testosterone in comparison to those who do not.

Bed-sharing may also affect the hormone secretions of the babies themselves. Research[22] has found that babies who bed-share in their first six months of life release less cortisol in a potentially stressful situation at twelve months of age. The scientists believe that this may be due to the positive effects on the baby's developing HPA-axis (see Chapter 1) and that bed-sharing may equip them with better stress responses than their non-bedsharing peers. These findings are echoed in research[23] that has found that babies who bed-share are significantly less likely to be obese when they are older than their solitary sleeping contemporaries. These findings may be due to the superior development of the HPA-axis and better emotional regulation and impulse control skills developed as a result of the nurturance received in babyhood, meaning that the bed-sharing babies were less likely to need to seek external emotional regulation via 'comfort eating' later in life and were able to control impulses to binge eat. Bed-sharing may also positively impact the development of the infant's brain, as discovered by research[24] that found that a history of bed-sharing in infancy was significantly associated with an increased level of cognitive competence at the age of six years.

Perhaps the most interesting potential benefit of bed-sharing is that it may in some way help to keep the baby safe at night. Research[25] has investigated the impact of the 'face to face' position most commonly adopted by bed-sharing mothers with their babies and the higher levels of carbon dioxide exhaled by the mothers into the baby's face. These increased levels of carbon dioxide may stimulate the baby to breathe and may help to protect the baby from SIDS. Similarly, the researchers theorised that this unique sleeping position may also prevent the baby from sleeping in the prone (tummy down) position, which may also protect them from SIDS. This is a point we will pick up again in the next chapter.

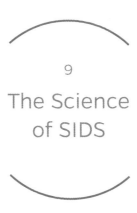

9

The Science of SIDS

Sudden Infant Death Syndrome (SIDS) terrifies all parents. This fear is enhanced by the lack of understanding, both public and professional, of the syndrome. Despite much research SIDS is still an enigma. The aetiology (cause) of SIDS continues to elude scientists. Theories come and go and small advances are made into potential understanding of the syndrome and possible ways to reduce the risk, but there are no definitive answers. SIDS is surrounded in much myth and misunderstanding, and many feel that efforts to reduce SIDS rates may inadvertently put some babies at risk, an issue touched on in the previous chapter in relation to co-sleeping.

SIDS accounts for just under ten per cent of all infant deaths. In the UK this amounts to around 300 babies per year, which equates to a rate of between 0.3 and 0.4 per 1,000 live births. Most SIDS cases occur under one year of age, but six per cent of cases occur in 12 to 24-month-olds. The formal definition of SIDS is the sudden and unexpected death of a baby under 12 months old for no immediately obvious reason.

For babies over 12 months old the term Sudden Unexplained Death is used. SIDS is more likely to affect baby boys and those who were born prematurely or at a low birth weight, though the reasons for this are unclear. The SIDS rate tends to peak in the colder months, with most deaths occurring in February, and the riskiest period in terms of age is between two and four months.

What is SIDS?

The label of SIDS is only given to explain a death after a post mortem has failed to find another cause of death. When the post mortem finds an explanation for the death, such as parental overlaying, asphyxiation or suffocation, then the cause of death is not recorded as SIDS. SIDS is therefore diagnosed by excluding other causes of death, rather than by recognising symptoms.

To this day nobody knows what causes SIDS. Scientists believe it is likely to be a combination of environmental and genetic factors, which somehow make a baby more vulnerable. SIDS appears to be characterised by a baby's failure to rouse during sleep cycles, which can occur during the night or day and wherever they are sleeping. Scientists believe that SIDS occurs in babies who have an undiagnosed pre-existing defect, which puts that particular baby at risk in certain environments, such as an unsafe sleeping environment, or when other factors are present, such as certain viruses or bacteria. The most prevalent theory about potential pre-existing defects is the possibility of abnormalities in the baby's brain stem and their serotonin pathways. Serotonin is an important neurotransmitter that regulates our important homeostatic systems, including sleep, heart rate, temperature and the ability to gasp for air, so it is easy to understand how an abnormality could lead to SIDS. Research[1] has shown that there are differences in the cells that are sensitive to serotonin in the brains of babies affected by SIDS, and that babies who have died from SIDS show abnormalities in their brain stem.[2] These are important findings, since the brain stem regulates both breathing and sleep, particularly in relation to serotonin pathways. To date, however, our understanding of any underlying pathophysiological aetiology of SIDS remains inadequate. We simply don't know what causes it.

Things that appear to increase the risk of SIDS

While the cause of SIDS remains unknown, there are many factors, both physical and environmental, which do appear to increase the risk. Understanding of risk factors is still inadequate, however, and many of the widely discussed risk factors are not quite so 'cut and dried' as many would believe. There are many opportunities for misunderstanding and misinformation, and generalised public health messages do little to improve matters.

Smoking

One of the most well understood and undisputed risk factors for SIDS is parental smoking. Research[3] has found that maternal smoking during pregnancy and maternal exposure to passive smoke increases the risk of SIDS significantly. What is less clear, however, is the effect of direct exposure to smoke post-birth. It is very hard to research the effects of smoke exposure on babies in terms of SIDS, as it is almost impossible to differentiate between the effects of smoking during pregnancy, including passive exposure, and smoke exposure after the birth. Those babies exposed to smoke post-birth are very likely to have been exposed to smoke in utero, whether the mother smoked herself or was exposed to passive smoke from a partner. This means it is not possible to ascertain the effect on SIDS risk of smoke exposure post-birth, as to do this scientists would need samples of mothers who didn't smoke during pregnancy and who also weren't exposed to any passive smoke, but did smoke post birth or had babies that were exposed to passive smoke. SIDS advice therefore extrapolates the effects of smoking during pregnancy and suggests that smoke exposure is a risk factor post-birth too.

Solitary sleeping

Research[4,5] has shown that babies sleeping in a different room to their parents are at greater risk of SIDS. In order to reduce the risk, babies should sleep in the same room as their parents for as long as possible; at least for the first six months. While co-sleeping in the same bedroom may be encouraged, however, most SIDS organisations discourage bed-sharing, claiming that it is unsafe. But as we have previously discussed, the standard message that 'the safest place for a baby to sleep is in their own cot, or similar container, in the parents' room for the first six months of life', does not give the full picture. To date there has been no research to support the claim that bed-sharing is unsafe in the absence of known risk factors and careful planning.

Formula feeding

It is a curious fact that all SIDS awareness promotion focusses on encouraging parents to breastfeed in order to reduce the risk of SIDS. Breastfeeding is said to have a protective effect. However, this isn't entirely true. The real correlation of interest between SIDS and infant feeding involves formula usage. According to research,[6] formula-fed babies have twice the risk of SIDS compared to those who are breastfed. Breastfeeding is normal for human babies; it doesn't offer special protection. As a deviation from the human norm, it is formula feeding that places babies at risk. This may seem like a pedantic distinction, but if parents are to make properly informed decisions, risks have to be discussed, as we have throughout the book, in terms of how the intervention (formula feeding, use of cots) compares with the normal (breastfeeding, sleeping with a parent).

Pillows and sleep surfaces

Research[7] has shown that using a pillow for babies under 12 months old increases the risk of SIDS by two and a half times. Similarly, loose blankets which may cover the head and cause overheating are also considered hazardous. Overly soft sleep surfaces are considered dangerous, hence the recommendation that mattresses are firm. What is less clear is how safe the new wave of 'baby surrounds' – soft pillow-like structures that parents use in cots to make babies feel cocooned and more secure – are. While these devices do seem to encourage a little more sleep, their safety in terms of SIDS risk is unknown. More worrying, however, is the use of these surrounds in the parental bed. Many parents use them as a way to feel that their baby is protected from overlaying in the parental bed. However, there is no evidence that the surrounds provide this protection, and in fact there is growing concern that their use may put babies at additional risk, as using them may mean that parents become complacent about other aspects of bed-sharing safety.

Prone sleeping

Most SIDS and public health organisations claim that prone (tummy) sleeping is one of the most important SIDS risks for parents to understand. There are many claims made about the efficacy of 'Back to Sleep' campaigns around the world, with claims of a six-fold reduction in SIDS deaths since the schemes were introduced in the early 1990s. While there is evidence that prone sleeping does present an increased risk, and all parents would be well advised to heed the advice to put their babies to sleep on their backs, there are some doubts about the true extent of the link between sleep position and SIDS.

The first important point to consider is the normality of tummy sleeping for babies. All mammals have a strong preference for sleeping on their front or side, perhaps in part to protect the body's most vulnerable area from predators during sleep. Until the last 25 to 30 years the human norm, particularly for babies, was to sleep in the same prone position as all other mammals. Human babies did not only spend their time asleep on their stomachs, however; they spent much more time prone during waking hours too. Before the invention of special baby seats, walkers, entertainment units, baby bouncers, rockers and travel systems, babies spent the majority of their time awake on their stomachs on the floor, in their parents' arms, or on a parent's back in a carrier with their bodies facing inwards, thus exercising the same important core muscles. Babies today spend very little time on their stomachs; so much so that health professionals advocate having special 'tummy time' to counter all the time babies spend on their backs, which delays physical development such as crawling and increases the risk of plagiocephaly (flat head syndrome). As babies spend less and less time on their stomachs and more and more time on their backs when awake, it follows that placing them on their stomachs to sleep may not be safe. What of the babies who spend their days on their stomachs, out of containers, though? The babies with strong core, head and neck strength? What of the babies who are always put to sleep on their stomachs and whose body strength, flexibility and frontal respiration capacity reflects this? Are they at the same risk? This is where the evidence is murky. In order to truly assess the risk of prone sleeping, researchers need to consider whether the tummy sleeping was planned and a normal and regular occurrence for the baby. Babies who have been put down on their stomach on a whim by an exhausted parent desperate to get their baby to sleep may be at a different risk than those put down on their fronts for all sleeps. Similarly, it is important to consider whether all babies are at risk from prone sleeping, or just those who have a pre-existing physiological condition which puts them at risk of SIDS.

There is no doubt that SIDS rates have fallen impressively since the introduction of 'Back to Sleep' campaigns in the early 1990s. There is doubt, however, about what actually caused this reduction in SIDS rates. Was it due to the 'Back to Sleep' campaigns, or was it an unrelated coincidence? SIDS rates had already started to fall in advance of the introduction of the campaigns. Would this trend have continued anyway? It is also possible that other variables played a role. The two most obvious are the rates of smoking and breastfeeding. Rates of maternal smoking during pregnancy have dramatically fallen over the last three decades, in line with increased SIDS awareness and health promotion. Could this have played a role in the decreasing SIDS rates? At the same time, breastfeeding rates rose. Interestingly, the rates of breastfeeding rose almost perfectly in line with the reduction in SIDS that is commonly attributed to 'Back to Sleep' education. Statistics from the Office for National Statistics Infant Feeding Surveys showed levels of breastfeeding exclusivity at birth rising from 60 per cent in 1990 to 66 per cent in 1995, 76 per cent in 2005 and 81 per cent in 2010. Over 20 per cent more mothers initiated breastfeeding in 2010 than in 1990. This was the same time period that saw SIDS rates fall dramatically. Is it possible that increased breastfeeding, along with reduced levels of maternal smoking, played a far bigger role in SIDS reduction than many organisations currently believe?

Over the last 25 to 30 years other changes have taken place in parenting, including a gradual reduction in too-early weaning and advice against dubious practices such as adding cereal to bottles. General public awareness of SIDS has risen greatly and parents are now much more aware of the guidelines about proper bedding and sleep environments, also thanks in part to the 'Back to Sleep' campaigns. Lastly, advances in medical science, which have led to differences in post-mortem diagnoses and the way deaths have been classified, may also have had an impact on SIDS rates.

Swedish neuroscientist Dr Nils Bergman[8] argues that the *'prone sleep position is the biological normative standard in healthy infants, supporting autonomic regulation'.* Bergman raises many questions about the potential stressor effect of placing babies to sleep on their backs, and the inhibited homeostatic capabilities that may occur as a result. He also examines the delayed neurodevelopment of babies who are placed to sleep on their backs, claiming that the current generalised advice may be detrimental to most babies, who are not predisposed to a greater risk of SIDS when sleeping in the prone position. Bergman argues that just because some babies might be saved by back sleeping, it should not become the normative sleeping practice for all.

The issue of tummy sleeping is now taboo, and while many parents still do it, they don't admit it to health professionals. Is the current blanket advice to 'never put a baby to sleep in the prone position' in fact more dangerous than sharing our understanding and the limitations of research with parents, and advising them to consider tummy sleeping only for a baby that spends plenty of time on their tummy and does so regularly during sleep, while minimising other risks? There are still many questions that need to be answered and we are a long way from having the full picture.

Not allowing the baby to suckle for comfort

Many professionals advise that dummy (pacifier) usage decreases the risk of SIDS, and this does appear to be backed up by research.[9] What is not understood, however, is the *mechanism* by which this works. Although research shows a correlation between dummy usage and reduced SIDS rates, nobody understands why. Is it really the *dummy itself* that helps, or the fact that the babies are being soothed by sucking? Sucking on a dummy for comfort may affect SIDS risk for two reasons: it decreases the baby's stress levels and lowers circulating cortisol, and may promote active sleep, in a similar way to breastfeeding. The real protective effect may not actually come from the dummy at all, but from the act of suckling and being comforted. Some babies may get this comfort from frequent night breastfeeding, while others, particularly if they are formula fed, may get the comfort they would not otherwise receive from a dummy.

Overheating

Scientists agree that overheating is a risk factor for SIDS. Research has shown[10,11,12] that high room temperature and too many blankets are potential risk factors for SIDS. What is not clear, however, is which specific temperatures should be avoided. Similarly, research cannot tell parents how much bedding is too much, what tog covering to use, or what the baby should wear underneath the bedding. While tables and charts exist showing parents what their baby should wear and what bedding they should have at any specific room temperature, these charts are not evidence-based. They are simply a matter of opinion. It is my personal opinion that many of these guides *underestimate* the clothing and tog rating of bedding that babies need to sleep in at night, meaning that babies may wake at night to seek parental heat as they are cold. Parents today are often paranoid about overheating their babies, perhaps in response to guidance given by health professionals or popular parenting books, and many may be unintentionally leaving their babies too cool at night. Aside from increased night waking, which may put babies at a higher risk of SIDS for other reasons, there has also been research[13] to show that babies who were too cold were also at an increased risk of SIDS. As with overheating, however, this really has not been researched enough.

Perhaps more alarming when it comes to non-evidence-based advice is the widespread recommendation of baby sleeping bags as a way to reduce the risk of SIDS. There is no evidence that baby sleeping bags reduce the risk of SIDS, which may surprise many parents and professionals! Research[14] has shown no difference in babies' body temperature when sleeping under blankets for an hour versus sleeping in a sleeping bag, and further research[15] has found no association between sleeping bag usage and SIDS rates.

Unsafe swaddling

The issue of swaddling is incredibly contentious. While there is no direct evidence that swaddling increases the risk of SIDS, there is some evidence that indicates that certain ways of swaddling may affect the baby's respiration and ability to arouse from sleep,[16, 17] which may contribute to SIDS. There are, however, ways in which swaddling can be practised that do not increase these risks. When swaddled, babies should always be placed to sleep on their backs. If parents want to swaddle their baby, they should do so as early as possible and should not begin to swaddle after ten weeks of age if they have not done so beforehand. They should stop swaddling as soon as the baby can roll and the swaddling should be done in such a way as not to compress the baby's chest, cover their head or overheat them. Just to confuse the issue even more, there is even some research[18] to suggest that if these rules are followed swaddling may even decrease the risk of SIDS.

Can breathing sensor monitors save babies?

There is no doubt that SIDS is a commercially viable business. Many companies manufacture breathing and sensor monitors designed to provide parents with peace of mind when it comes to their baby's sleep safety, and make lots of money from doing so. Unfortunately, however, there is no evidence that these monitors can help to decrease the risk of SIDS. Babies sadly can and do die with monitors in place. Of real concern is the potential for their use to actually *increase* the risk of SIDS! Parents may become complacent about SIDS risk factors if they use these monitors. They may ignore safe sleeping advice because they feel reassured by the presence of the monitor. While there is no doubt that these monitors can be useful if the baby is known to be at risk because of medical complications or prematurity, in most cases these expensive purchases provide parents with artificial peace of mind. This is why they are not generally recommended by professionals and SIDS organisations.

The way forward

It is clear that much more work needs to be done when it comes to understanding SIDS. In the meantime it is left to parents to navigate the minefield of information available. Unfortunately there is no simple rule to follow to protect babies from SIDS. At best, parents should try not to deviate from the human norm. We are not meant to feed our babies the milk of other species, to use lots of pillows, blankets and soft mattresses, to sleep in different rooms to our babies or to smoke around them. Any sleeping decisions made by parents should be informed and planned well in advance. Perhaps the most important message to take away when it comes to SIDS risks, however, is *not to make any rash decisions in a moment of exhaustion in the middle of the night*. Health professionals should be able to discuss sleep sensibly with parents, taking in each family's unique situation and risks and looking at how to reduce them. The current practice of 'one size fits all' SIDS advice often does not help families to make informed decisions, and as we have seen may even unintentionally put babies at risk.

10
The Scourge of Unwanted Sleep Advice and Criticism

Most parents, if left to their own devices, would likely parent their babies in the way science has found to be optimal. Parental instincts are strong. If babies cry we have an overwhelming urge to pick them up. If our arms are not enough to stem the tears, our instinct tells us to check for physical discomfort, including hunger. Even if they are not hungry, most babies are settled by suckling, particularly at the breast. These instincts are the same as those of all mammals. Mother monkeys, dogs and cats don't need parenting classes or specialists to give them advice about how to raise a healthy child, and neither do we. In many ways our constant quest for information and self-improvement is our downfall. In the world of parenting science things change quickly. One week researchers may announce that their study categorically proves that parents should do one thing, and the next week other researchers will proclaim the opposite. Advice is ever-changing and ever-confusing. The more confused parents become, the harder they find it to listen to their instincts and the more they question their innate ability to raise their child. In a world without parenting advice there would probably be a lot more great parents and happy children.

Baby sleep advice is everywhere: everyone is an expert, from the scientific researchers to a stranger in a coffee shop. They all have an opinion, and most people believe that their way is 'the right way'! All this advice, both expert and not so expert, tends to besiege new parents whether they ask for it or not. Just as pregnancy is full of unwanted predictions of gender, date of birth and birth weight, new parenthood is full of unwanted suggestions for how to improve the little darling's sleep, whether the parent feels their baby has a sleeping problem or not. Occasionally the advice is helpful, but far more often it is confusing, disempowering and guilt-inducing. Just as these mothers found:

> 'There is so much societal pressure for training your baby to sleep without you.'

> 'I breastfed my little girl and fed her often when she woke in the night. Several of my friends scolded me for creating this bad night-time habit.'

> 'My sister told me my parenting style will mean my child will never be independent and that he should be going to sleep alone without me cuddling him.'

> 'Hearing other people's opinions made me feel like I was going against 'the rules'.'

> 'I've been told numerous times that I've made a rod for my own back by rocking, cuddling and feeding to sleep, which made me feel guilty.'

'A lot of people have made me feel guilty, my husband being one of them. At one point he blamed my son's sleep on me, saying I have mollycoddled him.'

'At our seven-month review the health visitor said that my baby would become 'needy' if I continued feeding her to sleep and that I must teach her to self-settle.'

'Some family have said that perhaps our daughter doesn't sleep through the night because she's still in our room past 6 months.'

'My health visitor said that I've 'made a rod for my own back' by having my daughter in my bed and that it wasn't safe. I breastfeed and have a bedside cot.'

'I was made to feel guilty for letting my baby sleep on the breast. The general consensus out there is that I shouldn't allow this, so that he can learn to settle himself.'

'Everyone tries to convince me that our bed-sharing is setting us up for failure.'

When it comes to sleep advice from healthcare professionals, a worrying trend emerges. While there are undoubtedly many wonderful health visitors, midwives, GPs and paediatricians, who focus on giving current, evidence-based, unbiased sleep advice, there are also many who give advice based on their own personal opinion and experience. Sometimes this advice is totally unsolicited and given to parents who have not even mentioned concerns about their child's sleep.

While researching this book I asked over 200 parents if they had ever received any unsolicited and unwanted baby sleep advice. A huge 86 per cent answered yes. Of these, 31 per cent indicated they had received the advice from a family doctor or nurse, such as a health visitor; 69 per cent said that they had received unsolicited and unwanted baby sleep advice from friends and family; and ten per cent reported that they had received unsolicited and unwanted baby sleep advice from complete strangers. In the overwhelming majority of cases the sleep advice given involved 'cry based' sleep training, including 'controlled crying' or 'cry it out' methods. Almost 70 per cent of healthcare professionals advised parents to leave their babies to cry for a set period of time in order to 'teach them to self-settle'; the remaining 25 per cent of medical professionals advised parents to make sure the baby slept alone in order to not form 'bad habits' and advised cutting down on night feeds. Less than five per cent of healthcare professionals gave advice that could be seen as 'baby friendly' and evidence-based. This is particularly shocking when you consider that most of this advice was unwanted and unsolicited by the parents in question.

How to handle unwanted sleep advice from a health professional

Hopefully you will be one of the lucky ones and encounter healthcare providers who keep their knowledge of infant sleep up to date and maintain evidence-based practice. Unfortunately it is not always possible to know if your provider fits into this category in advance of meeting them, so preparing a few simple stock responses to any advice they may give you regarding your baby's sleep can help you to feel more in control of the situation. Consider replying using the following examples:

1. 'That's interesting. Please can you provide me with a reference to some research that supports your suggestion, so that I can take a read for myself and investigate further?'

2. 'Thank you for your suggestion. I will consider it when I do my own research and let you know what I decide to do.'

3. 'Thank you for trying to help. However, we are happy with how things are at the moment.'

4. 'Can you tell me what the risks and benefits are to my baby of this approach please?'

5. 'Thank you for your advice. Is this your personal belief or is it evidence based?'

Remember that if you are unhappy with the information given to you by your healthcare provider, you are perfectly within your rights to ask to see a different one. If the advice you receive is particularly non-evidence-based and outdated, you may also consider making a formal complaint. This isn't nice to do, but in many cases is the best way to try to prevent other new parents falling prey to poor advice in the future. Sometimes change in services is best led from the ground up, especially if top-down monitoring of services is not particularly effective.

How to handle unwanted sleep advice from a friend or relative

In many ways responding to unwanted baby sleep advice from friends and relatives is harder than dealing with health professionals. While it can sometimes be hard to question information provided by somebody in a position of authority, it is often much harder when that person is somebody you know and love. Most parents wouldn't be particularly concerned about damaging their relationship with a healthcare professional. If advice from a health professional jars it is relatively easy to avoid seeing that person again, but the same is not true of friends and family.

In most cases friends and family give unsolicited sleep advice because they care. They see their friends, sisters, daughters, brothers and sons looking exhausted and stressed and they want to help. You would probably feel the same if the situation was reversed. If friends and family have had their own children, they likely found a method that worked for them to get more sleep and they naturally want to share it. If they are yet to have children of their own they probably have strong opinions about what does and doesn't work. These are likely to be very naïve!

In most cases the advice is well meant, however much you may disagree with it, and it can be helpful to keep this in mind. In particular family and friends may give advice that they know to be at odds with your current parenting style, and they may even criticise the way you are parenting. Again this is likely to be because they believe that what you are doing currently isn't working. They may think that the way you parent at night is causing the 'sleep problems' that leave you looking and feeling so exhausted. Thus they criticise your choices if they feel that they are responsible for your current predicament. This is particularly true if the advice comes from a friend or family member who parented a few decades ago, when parenting styles were very different and before science had investigated baby sleep. It must be confusing for a friend and family member to see a loved one suffering when they think that they know 'the answer', and to see their helpful (in their eyes!) suggestions ignored.

When responding to unwanted parenting advice from friends and family, you must consider the effect of your words on those giving the advice. If the advice comes from somebody who is a parent there is a high chance that you may offend them by dismissing or criticising their suggestions, which will seem to them as criticism of their own parenting decisions. While up-to-date research may show the damaging effects of the methods they suggest, be careful how you explain this to them, as you may cause them to feel guilty. After all, nobody likes to learn that the way they have raised a child might have put them at risk or been less than optimal. If you are sensitive, and lucky, you may find that your friend or family member is open to hearing about the latest research and may even use it in future to inform their parenting or grandparenting. However, it takes a strong person to realise, admit and even forgive themselves for past mistakes. For many the new knowledge may result in 'cognitive dissonance'. This is a state of mind in which it is too painful to hear information that conflicts with a deeply held belief or previous practice, which causes the person to try to subconsciously attack the new information to lessen the psychological unease that they feel. Hearing that leaving a baby to cry can have long-term negative consequences can be incredibly painful for somebody who has left a baby to 'cry it out' to hear. So if the person giving the advice experiences cognitive dissonance, they are likely to attack the idea that 'cry it out' is damaging, criticising the research, belittling the experts and uttering the infamous phrase 'well, it never did me/my baby any harm'. This complete dismissal of information that conflicts with their deeply held beliefs is in fact a complicated psychological protection mechanism, and one that is very hard to get around. Overcoming cognitive dissonance requires empathy, understanding, support and patience. Simply referencing the research papers, books, blogs and magazine articles is likely to drive the person further into a state of dissonance. Waiting, empathising and slowly drip-feeding new information, at times when the person may be more receptive, is far more likely to be successful at changing opinions.

It is worth practising and memorising a couple of stock responses to friends and family members when they recommend something that is completely against your parenting beliefs. Reply in a calm, warm but very assertive manner, which makes it clear that you are not open to further discussion at that time. The following suggestions may help you to think about what to say the next time you receive unsolicited and unwanted baby sleep advice:

'Thanks so much for thinking of us. I'll have a think about what you've said and discuss it with my partner/health visitor/doctor.'

'That's really interesting, thanks for letting me know. I'll do some more research on that later.'

'Thanks for your suggestions. I think we're OK with how things are at the moment, but it's something we'll maybe consider in the future.'

'It's really interesting to hear how you handled things with your own children. They are all so different aren't they?'

'Thanks for your help. We've decided on a very specific way of parenting and that doesn't quite fit with what we do.'

'Isn't it confusing how quickly research and understanding changes? That's not something that is recommended anymore.'

Finally, keep reminding yourself why you are choosing to parent in the way that you are, especially when advice may make you question your choices. Keep focussed on the long term, and if possible surround yourself with as many like-minded parents as possible. This may be in real life, or online. These kindred spirits are the ones who will help you to stay confident in your choices and provide the support you need to keep going. Sometimes it may be wise to distance yourself for a while from those in 'real life' who undermine and make you question your choices, until you feel stronger. Having top-up sessions of like-minded positivity from other parents is one of the keys to sticking to a gentle night-time parenting path, particularly when those around you have very different points of view.

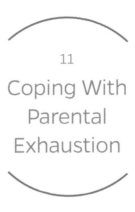

11

Coping With Parental Exhaustion

There is no doubt about it: parenting a baby and young child is utterly exhausting. The days are a relentless round of feeding, calming tears, entertaining and cleaning up various bodily fluids. The cycle continues at night, with only a few hours of peace if you are lucky. There are no days off, no breaks, no sick leave. Weekends no longer offer the rest and respite they once did. Holidays present more challenges and often more stress than staying at home. Life as you knew it has gone, never to be the same again. Lazy Saturday lie-ins and Sunday afternoon naps are a thing of the past. Life becomes monotonous and drains every ounce of energy from you. You may get a cute co-worker whose smiles make you feel prouder and happier than any bonus cheque, but that doesn't stop most parents from reaching depths of desperation that they never previously thought possible. It is in precisely these depths of desperation that the 'sleep trainers' lurk, in the darkness where parents leave their instincts and common sense behind and agree to do things that they never would during their more lucid, calmer moments.

Should new parents make themselves martyrs and run themselves into the ground for the sake of their babies? Is the only solution to 'wait it out', no matter what the cost to the mother's mental and physical health? Of course not. Maternal health matters just as much as infant health. The real goal of the family is to create happy babies and happy mummies, not one at the expense of the other. Happy mothers are ones who take care of themselves and their needs as much as possible, while also meeting the needs of their babies.

What is your role?

If the role of 'mother' had a job description, what would it include?

- To discover and care for all physical needs of the baby, including feeding, keeping clean, keeping warm, getting to sleep, meeting any medical needs and providing support for developing skills.
- To discover and care for all emotional needs of the baby, including soothing and calming, entertaining, allowing the baby's dependency and allowing them to express emotions while providing external regulation and containment.
- To provide a safe and 'baby friendly' environment during the day and at night.
- To provide protection for the baby against any potential harm, both physical and emotional.
- To engage in appropriate self-care so that you can provide all of the above to the baby. This includes (but is not limited to): eating nutritious food to ensure adequate daily calorie intake, drinking enough water, catching up on sleep where and when possible in order to meet the needs of the baby during the night, seeking external support as and when necessary, and finding outlets for emotional and physical needs.

Hours: Twenty-four hours per day, seven days per week
Holiday: None
Sick Pay: None
Contract: Permanent, indefinite length
Remuneration: None (but plenty of love and gummy smiles)

Would the job description also include working outside the home, voluntary work, meal preparation, laundry and housework? Some may feel it does, but these tasks are actually extraneous to mothering. Other work may sometimes be necessary to provide financially for the baby, and some degree of housework is necessary to provide a safe environment. Similarly some laundry and food preparation is necessary. Is it necessary, however, to provide this for all other members of the household? Many mothers fall into the trap of feeling that because they are now staying at home, some permanently, some temporarily, that they should take on the lion's share of the household chores, especially if their partners work full-time outside of the home. This extra work is not a core part of mothering, however. It is outside of the job description. Why should mothers take it on just because they may be the ones at home all day? The primary role of motherhood is taking care of the child, which also requires self-care on behalf of the mother to enable her to meet the child's needs. Any other work that needs doing in the house should be shared by all who live there. No job in the world is more demanding than mothering, and indeed no job is more important. Women should not feel the need to take on anything else. Mothering is enough. It is more than enough.

Mindfulness and gratitude

When you are sleep-deprived and exhausted it becomes all too easy to slip into a downward spiral of negative thinking.

It may seem as if you will never get a full night's sleep again. You may have forgotten what it felt like to feel energetic. The days of having freshly washed hair and clean clothes may seem like a distant memory. There may be days when you focus on just how much of 'you' you have lost: the confident career woman, the runner or gym goer, the reliable friend, the enthusiastic lover, the helper, the one in control, the one who was never late, the one who always had manicured nails and neatly applied make-up. Whoever you were before having a baby you are no longer and may never be again. In some sense new motherhood is also a time for mourning. Mourning your past life and who you once were. New motherhood is a time of transition. For some that transition is easy; they triumphantly shed their previous skin and don their new outfit with aplomb. Others may cling on to their old skin, reluctant to let it go, not sure if the new one is really for them, reluctantly trying it on for size and not liking what they see in the mirror. This transition is doubtless made harder when seen through dry, blood-shot, exhausted eyes. The less we like what we see in the mirror, the harder it is to accept it and the more we focus on our problems, the harder it becomes to see our way out of the darkness.

Meeting motherhood with gratitude, even at times when we may feel at our least grateful, can be an immensely powerful way to cope with the transition and to navigate the darkest depths of sleep deprivation. Being mindful and focussing on just the present moment in time and all of the wonders that it brings, without fretting about yesterday or worrying about tomorrow, holds the key to happier new parenthood. For many this way of thinking does not come easily. We live in a hyper-critical society where flaws are all too quickly pointed out. We spend too long analysing our mistakes and worrying about our future. We rarely live in 'the now' or take time to count our many blessings. Often we don't notice them until they are gone.

Becoming grateful as a new parent means simply noticing what you have in the present moment and looking for and appreciating the good. Waking tired at 5am means that you are awake to greet a new day and have been woken by one of the greatest gifts in the world – a healthy child. Struggling to get out of bed with exhaustion means that you are lucky enough to have a bed, with warm coverings in a safe and secure house. Being woken at 2am to feed a baby means that you are able to respond to your child's need for nourishment. There are always positives, always things to be grateful for. Focusing on these may be difficult at first, but can produce a tremendous mind-shift.

Being mindful as a parent means focusing on the here and now. It means that yesterday has passed. There is no use fretting over something that you did or didn't do. What you did yesterday has happened: you cannot change it, you can only learn from it and move on. Tomorrow hasn't happened yet, and you cannot control something that will happen tomorrow. Worrying about the future will not – cannot – change it. It will only make you stressed and anxious. Worrying about going back to work and how your baby will settle in daycare does nothing to change the outcome, but it will take the joy out of today. Fretting about your baby's ability to sleep without your constant presence in three months' time is fruitless. In three months everything will be different: you cannot possibly predict what life will be like then, so what is the use in trying? It will only take the joy out of today. Parent the baby you have today. You have already parented yesterday's baby and tomorrow's baby does not exist yet. Focus on making it through minute by minute. Focus on your baby's current needs, because they are the only needs there are and the only ones that matter. Becoming a more mindful parent takes an enormous pressure off. When you realise that all you can do is focus on what you do today and doing your best, the tension of worrying about the long-term dissipates. You learn to enjoy yourself and parent without fear of doing wrong, creating bad habits or feeling guilty. In turn the weight of the pressure you subconsciously place upon yourself lifts and everything becomes lighter, easier and more enjoyable.

Emergency oxygen

If you are feeling at the end of your tether with your baby's sleep it is vitally important that you get help. That help can look different for different people. For some the help may be in the shape of a phone call to a best friend, a visit from their mother, a date night with their partner, a massage, a long bath, exercise or reading a book. How you cope doesn't really matter: the important thing is that you notice that you need a break and you somehow make it happen.

Consider this analogy: the safety announcement on commercial airlines. Flight attendants instruct that in the event of an emergency requiring oxygen masks, those travelling with young children should fix their own masks first before helping their children. If you pass out from lack of oxygen while fitting your child's mask, you will not be able to help them when the plane makes an emergency landing. Thus fitting your own oxygen mask first is not selfish, it is a necessity. This isn't an excuse for parenting selfishly; it is the key to parenting sensibly. Sometimes you must put your own needs first in order to protect your baby.

Why crying in arms is not the same as sleep-training

Conventional sleep-training relies on babies crying themselves to sleep until they no longer cry for their parents.

The babies learn that their parents do not respond to their cries, so they stop communicating and ultimately stop crying. This has given crying a bad name. Many parents are afraid to allow their babies to cry at all, or find it too difficult to do so. Many fathers in particular find that they are unable to soothe their babies, and that their baby may cry in their arms for half an hour or more, but stop crying instantly when the mother holds them, particularly if she is breastfeeding. This can lead to partners feeling disempowered. They are unable to stop their baby crying so they rarely try, instead passing the child to the mother. Crying in the arms of a loving parent, however, is nothing like leaving a baby crying alone in a cot. If all the baby's physical needs have been met: they are not hungry, their nappy is clean, they are comfortable and not ill, then there is no harm in them being cradled in the arms of a loving parent who is fully present and engaging and empathising with the baby, even if they continue to cry. The role of the parent in this moment is to provide all the comfort and presence they can and to support the baby, even though the baby may be crying. If the mother is present and able to comfort the baby this of course is always preferable, but if she is not present, or she needs to rest and to take time away from the baby in order to get some 'emergency oxygen' to be a better mother, then there is no harm to the baby from crying 'in arms' for a while.

Is your exhaustion solely due to your baby's sleep?

While there is no doubt that new parenting is exhausting, for some mothers in particular there may be other things at play. It is always important to rule out physical causes of exhaustion, particularly the following:

Inadequate food and water intake

The postnatal period is not the time to diet. Breastfeeding

mothers should consume around 1,800 calories per day. Eating well is incredibly important to stay healthy and to have adequate energy to care for the baby. Similarly drinking adequate fluid is vital. The easiest way to tell if you are drinking enough is by monitoring the colour of your urine: it should be a very pale straw colour. If it is darker you are dehydrated and need to drink more.

Postpartum thyroiditis

Postpartum thyroiditis affects around 5 per cent of new mothers, although it is commonly misunderstood and under-diagnosed by medical professionals. After birth the thyroid may become over- or underactive, or even both. A common pattern is for hyperthyroidism (overactive) to be followed by hypothyroidism (underactive). The onset of thyroid problems usually comes between two and six months post-partum, when parents are often struggling with sleep deprivation. Symptoms can include tiredness, lack of energy, depression, memory problems and general aches and pains, which are generally dismissed as normal for new parenthood.

Postpartum depression and birth trauma

Postpartum depression (PPD), sometimes known as postnatal depression (PND), affects around a fifth to a quarter of all new mothers. Symptoms can include tiredness, lack of energy, feelings of low self-esteem and low self-worth, guilt, lack of enjoyment in life, problems bonding with the baby and changes in eating and sleeping habits. PPD is incredibly common and a lot of support is available, but diagnosis is sometimes hard and women can be left undiagnosed, causing them to suffer unnecessarily.

Feelings arising from the birth can also cause difficulties in the early months and years of parenthood. There is no one definition of a traumatic birth: what may seem like 'a good birth' to some may prove to be deeply traumatic to others. Traumatic births can be natural or they can be surgical. One important factor, however, seems to be how 'in control' the parents felt during the experience. Birth trauma can take the enjoyment out of parenting and cause problems for many years to come if it remains undiagnosed and untreated. For this reason any unresolved feelings about the birth should always be discussed with a specially trained birth afterthoughts counsellor or support organisation.

Iron deficiency

Many new mothers are iron deficient. For some this may be as a direct result of blood loss related to birth, while others may be anaemic for no obvious reason. If a woman starts pregnancy with lowered iron stores these will be depleted during the pregnancy, leaving her deficient after birth even if she had no excessive bleeding. Iron deficiency can cause symptoms that mothers put down to tiredness from looking after a sleepless baby, and is also linked to an increased risk of PPD, lowered milk production, fatigue, exhaustion and an increased frequency of urinary tract infections.

Magnesium and zinc deficiency

It is estimated that over half of adults are currently deficient in the trace mineral magnesium and a similar number may be deficient in zinc. Magnesium and zinc appear to play a key role in many neurological processes and their role in depression is well known. Research[1] has shown that magnesium may play a significant role in PPD and a similar study also implicates zinc.[2] Magnesium and zinc deficiencies can also cause headaches, exhaustion, muscular pain and cramps, sleeping disturbances and lowered immunity.

Vitamin B12 deficiency

Postpartum vitamin B12 deficiency is common, yet under-diagnosed. It is estimated that around a quarter of all adults are deficient in vitamin B12, which is commonly known as the energy-giving vitamin. Deficiency of B12 may result in extreme tiredness and lethargy, irritability and depression, pins and needles, sores in the mouth or on the tongue and 'brain fog'.

It is not a given that new parenthood must be full of exhaustion and negative feelings. If you feel that any of these may apply to you it is important that you seek appropriate advice from someone well qualified. It may seem a strange idea that parents should look at their own health and behaviour in order to better cope with their baby's sleep, but it can be hugely beneficial.

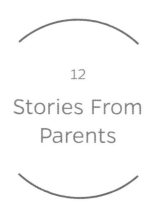

12

Stories From Parents

The final chapter of this book is dedicated entirely to the real baby sleep experts: parents themselves. In this chapter a selection of parents share their baby sleep journeys, from their developing understanding of their babies' needs to how they dealt with unhelpful advice. I would like to thank all of the parents who have shared their stories with me. I hope you find them as interesting and inspiring as I did.

'When we had just had our little man we planned to co-sleep with him in our room (but not in our bed) as advised by the midwives. Soon we came to find that our little man didn't want to sleep in any container, only in our arms. I breastfeed and we decided to let him sleep with us, not only because he so desperately seemed to need it, but also because it meant more sleep for me as he could feed while sleeping. Our choices seemed to go against all advice from professionals, but we followed our intuition and it meant a happy baby and a happy mummy. Crying raises my stress levels enormously, I absolutely cannot

listen to my little man crying, it makes me on edge and always has done. If crying gives me so much stress, it must be horrible for my baby, especially in a brain that develops so much and so quickly. I must admit I thought I would follow all conventional advice from 'childcare professionals', but that advice went against my natural instincts and common sense, so I didn't. My baby feels safe close to me, during the day and during the night. That is how nature intended motherhood and that is how babies thrive and gain their confidence. I know it is much easier if you know how to live in the moment, so that would be something to learn first, but my son and I have the most beautiful bond and I don't regret any choices we made.'

'I've been bed-sharing and wearing my six-month-old to sleep since she was a few weeks old. I could have saved so much money on the cot and co-sleeper if only I'd known. I'm a first-time mum and I was not expecting the bone tiredness that is ever present and unrelenting. I would definitely say we got a non-sleeper. Coping is hard and sometimes you don't. Bed-sharing helps us to get more sleep. I cannot imagine how much worse it would be to actually get out of bed every time the baby wakes. It feels natural to respond to her cries, although I do feel pressure from friends and family to 'let her cry a bit' or sleep train. We tried patting her to sleep in her cot at six weeks old on the advice of child health nurses, it was horrible. She'd scream until she fell asleep (for up to an hour) and then only sleep for thirty minutes. I think we tried for two days and my partner and I said 'Forget this!'. Sleep is still unpredictable at six months, but it's better than the early days. In those days you just survive. Now we live a little! I will breastfeed and bed-share as long as she needs because I'm her mum and that's how we roll. But I'm sort of looking forward to the day she's in her own room when I can sleep all night and throw these bras with the little clips in the bin! I'm under no illusions that it will be any time soon, but that's OK. One day.'

'We chose to bed-share because... actually, we didn't choose it, we just followed our instincts. Both our girls were on the small side when they were born and it felt wrong to put them down in a crib or cot. They spent the first couple of months on either me or my husband. We then moved them onto a mattress next to us. Our older daughter slept with us until she was three and then moved into her bedroom with no problems or fuss at all. She knows that she can still sleep with us whenever she wants or needs to though. Our second baby is nine months old and even though she still doesn't sleep through the night, most nights I don't even know when, or for how long, she is awake as she finds my breast and drifts back to sleep without disturbing me much.'

'The decision to sleep with my baby came as I wanted to enhance my milk production so I kept her skin-to-skin in the hospital and then she slept on my chest till she was almost four months. We went to visit my parents in Spain and single-handedly she made the decision to sleep by my side from then on. It also became the only way to sleep for me. If I tried to put her in a cot she'd be crying and then wake up more often too. Sleep training does not agree with me. I have taken unpaid leave until she turns ten months old to dedicate my time to her. I would rather listen closely to her needs, instead of dictating foreign routines to both of us. Breastfeeding at night has helped me sleep even though it sounds paradoxical. I don't know the science behind it but it's true. I don't even feel her latching on and sometimes I can't remember how many times she feeds at night. To make a little more room in the bed, we have sidecarred the unused cot we bought and sometimes she is there for naps and I lie beside *her while I nurse her to sleep, but some nights it's me mostly in the cot! I don't really like giving advice to new moms because if I have learnt something from this experience it is this: listen and be grateful for all the stories but first and foremost listen to your baby and to yourself. You're right more often than not.'*

'As a professional working with families I see a lot of parents struggle with what everyone else is doing and saying, when what they really want to do is bed down with their babies and forget the world. I just ask people to do what feels right for their own families, and that the path of least resistance, in terms of being responsive and loving, actually means you get more sleep and you end up with very strong, supported, independent and confident children. They know who's got their back from dot. And it makes a huge difference. Most of the emotional work I end up doing with older kids with separation anxiety and developmental social issues are kids of parents who did lots of harsh sleep training and have attachment issues.'

'My baby was the only one on the postnatal ward who wouldn't sleep in the little plastic boxes, so he fed and slept on me all night. When we got home we spent a few nights trying to get him to sleep in a Moses basket with no luck and I was up in a chair most of the night feeding anyway so no one got any sleep. My mum suggested feeding him lying down and keeping him in the bed and for the first time in days I had more than a snatched ten minutes of sleep here and there. After much googling I realised how normal and natural it is for human babies to want to sleep and feed this way and reassured myself that my little one would definitely have been a survivor in caveman days. In time I was able to snooze through night feeds and we were both comfortable and content and knew what we were doing so that helped massively to catch up with sleep.

My son is now almost sixteen months old. Sleep has massively improved but we still have periods where he doesn't sleep so well. He never liked a cot and so we got him a toddler bed at just over a year and he has now done several nights completely in his own bed with only a few wake ups for his dummy or a cuddle. I still bring him in our bed if he doesn't settle quickly as it's the quickest way for everyone to get back to sleep. I have memories of getting into my parents bed if I woke in the night at around five or six and feeling very comforted by that and I want my son to feel the same for as long as he needs.'

'When my son's eczema developed, we didn't really know much about skin conditions. We knew he was itchy and rashy but the journey his dietary-related eczema problems (and, at that stage, unknown allergies) took us on had yet to unravel itself. All we knew was that we had a baby who went from sleeping four to five hour stretches as a newborn to forty-five minute stretches as a three-month-old. When his sleep regressed, we had a lot of bad advice about how to make him sleep longer, including being told that he's hungry, he's sleeping too much during the day, he needs to be left alone to cry and self soothe, etc. I wish I'd trusted my instincts. I wish I'd trusted my baby. He wasn't 'being naughty' and 'not giving Mummy a break'. He was communicating to us that his body was uncomfortable, he was itchy and suffering from allergic reactions. Instead I gave into the bad advice and allowed formula. I started him on solids too early and left him to cry all alone once, though I scooped him up before he cried himself to sleep. After a couple of months of sleep deprivation, tears and sheer exhaustion, I had a moment. I said to my husband, 'We just have to accept that he isn't going to sleep'. This was a game-changer for us! From this realisation we stopped fighting it and were able to go with it. This enabled us to start focusing on our son's needs, day* or night, instead of focusing on the time of night or how many times we'd gotten out of bed. We got on with it, we supported each other and we drank a lot of coffee! My son needed a 2am bath and full body wet wraps every morning. We did it. He needed to co-sleep so that we could hold his limbs down to stop him rubbing at his body. We did it. He needed to be rocked or fed to sleep so that he felt safe, comfortable, distracted and so he knew that even though his physical body was always itchy and sore, Mummy loves him. Mummy is always there for him and will help him. My baby never cried for no reason or refused sleep because he was being naughty. I will never regret holding and cuddling my baby. Before you know it, they're not babies anymore. He is twenty months old now. His eczema and allergies are well managed through diet and focusing on gut health. He is still rocked to sleep and he still co-sleeps. We love it! I learned a lot from his first year. Now my advice to any new mum is to trust your instincts, you know more than you think you do.'

'A great piece of advice I received was 'Do whatever works!'. It's simple, but in the often judgemental, opinionated, advice-saturated world of parenting it is respectful of the fact that every baby is different, every parent is different, every situation is different, and you need to do what works for you and your baby. 'Whatever works' for me was having baby in a sling in the day, breastfeeding to sleep and bed-sharing at night. I never felt like I was 'spoiling the baby', because it is biologically normal for an infant to want to be close to their mum, to wake and feed at night. We chose not to sleep train because it would be stressful for us both to fight what is natural and I saw no benefit in doing so. We both get plenty of sleep at night, and six months in I can honestly say there have only been a handful of sleepless nights in the whole journey. I'm not sure if this is because I have been blessed with a 'good sleeper', or whether he sleeps well because he is secure and confident that his needs will always be met. One day he will move into his cot, but we are just going to play it by ear.'

'The best thing that we found was having a family bedtime from day one. Our baby naturally had a late bedtime of around eleven o'clock at night, so we all went to bed together (he slept in the cot next to me). He also got up later. During maternity leave I went to bed at the same time as him, breastfed through the night and we both woke later in the morning. As time went on we slowly moved his bedtime further forward to fit with our day routines. He is now eleven months and his bedtime is 8:30pm. Having a family bedtime and later bedtime I feel has maximized my potential sleep and has helped me continue breastfeeding through the night. Since going back to work he goes to sleep and I now continue working if I have to until his next feed. He still sleeps next to me in his cot and we sometimes have sleepy cuddles in the night.'

'The best advice I had was to see it as a blessing. Because of breastfeeding I was the only one able to see to them and spend that time feeding them and every time that should be considered a blessing. I have twins and decided that co-sleeping would be too awkward, so they were in Moses baskets next to me until they were bigger and then went into a cotbed together with the side off next to my bed. I started off tandem feeding and waking the other when one woke, but realised that this wasn't fair on them, so I have been feeding each baby on demand at night with as little fuss as possible to avoid stirring the other. It's hard going as some bad nights have involved being up half a dozen times per baby! However, they have their own patterns of waking now and I'm glad that I didn't keep forcing them to feed at the same time.'

'Our experiences with baby number two were hard. We made the decision with our first daughter never to do sleep training or controlled crying, but she was one of those unusual babies who was happier sleeping spread out in her own cot. She always slept for fairly long stretches between feeds and other than a few periods of unsettled sleep she had always been easy in terms of sleep. Then we had our second daughter. She was quite small at birth and it was clear from the start that she needed to catch up. She fed constantly and hated being put down. Out of sheer exhaustion we started bed-sharing. She woke very frequently but if I fed her immediately she would quieten down and go back to sleep. She loved being close to us and liked to sleep with her hand touching my face or my husband's. It wasn't easy. I thought I could manage sleep deprivation as my job involves shift work, but this was like a shift that never finished! We worked out a system where my husband would look after both girls in the morning at the weekend so I didn't get too far behind with sleep, and he would also take the baby from 5am (when she woke) so I could get another hour or so before our older child woke. It was hard, but worth it to see how jolly, contented and settled she was. Gradually it got easier, but mainly we adapted to the baby rather than making our sweet, happy baby adapt to us. Now she starts the night in her cot and comes into our bed when she wakes, but now we even miss her when she's in her cot!'

'I was very naive about baby sleep when I had my daughter, not realising that she might need some help to get to sleep. However, under the guidance of my mother and with the ongoing support of my husband we have muddled through the first nine months of parenthood. We bed-share and I breastfeed her to sleep for all her naps and when she stirs during the night. It has meant I'm not getting up and getting cold when she decides that she wants boobies! Also she gets cuddled all night, which is exactly how I love to sleep! My mum parented me the same way and she just says to me she was a lazy parent! I have tried to keep the mantra of 'she'll do it when she's ready' in my mind in regard to her sleeping through. We have turned our bedroom into a campsite and my daughter and I share the queen-size bed while my husband gets a full night's sleep on the single bed! He doesn't even wake to the baby now. Since we have slept like this we are all getting the rest we need. A friend tried to tell me that when I return to work I'll have to have 'a few hard nights to get her to sleep the entire night'. Fortunately, as we continue on this journey, I've gotten better at not taking these comments to heart and just having confidence in my intuition as to how we parent our child. I suppose what I've learned over the last few months is that you do what's right for your baby and your family. No one else has the complete story and they don't know your baby as well as you. A friend told me that you keep doing what works and then when it doesn't work anymore you change it. So that's what I'm trying to do.'

'When I was pregnant I found out that I had to have a caesarean delivery due to complete placenta praevia. This was far from my birth plan so I had a difficult time accepting that my son would enter this world in a cold, sterile room. After much thought and research with my midwife we were able to agree on a family-centred caesarean. This allowed my son to feel the most comfortable as soon as possible. We wanted him to not lose his comforts, which had been hearing my heartbeat and voice, and feeling warm and full, just to name a few. As soon as he was placed next to me in the operating room my son stopped crying. There was no doubt that being with his momma made him feel comfortable in a world that was so new to him. Because of that experience, I wanted for him to be near me all the time, which immediately altered any parenting ideas I had beforehand. We tried out many baby carriers until we agreed on a ring sling that we love. If he's not sleeping in the sling, we're always found snuggling together on our family bed. This wasn't the plan, but I am so happy that his birth experience forced me to view life through his eyes. Today at almost six months old he is a happy baby, as long as momma is holding him or nearby, and I'm more than happy with that!'

'When we got home after the birth I really struggled with my son's sleep. My father had built an amazing sidecar so he could have his own sleep surface inches from me and my husband and I had spent months curating a beautiful nursery for him to nap in during the day. Baby had other plans though. He struggled to fall and stay asleep and only did so on my chest for weeks. Any attempt to move him off me woke him immediately. A few weeks in I was able to get him to sleep in his stroller or being worn on walks during the day, and Dad would occasionally have luck walking him down, but by and large it was on me. I had dreams of a TV baby. I imagined I would nurse him drowsy and lay him down and watch him peacefully drift off while I got to do adult stuff for a few hours. I dreamed of the day he would sleep anywhere by himself and start the night alone so I could have my body back and enjoy a moment with my husband on the couch. We are now seven months in and none of those things have happened. I nurse him through every nap. I go to bed with him at six o'clock every night and am available for comfort sucking every minute of the night. It's the hardest thing I have ever done. The unrelenting nature of his needs is beyond anything I imagined. But when I think of the look on his face when I would try to unlatch him and lay him down, going from peaceful, perfectly sleepy baby to wide awake and fearful, I know that however hard it is for me it is *worth it to be there for my guy. My friends and family think I'm crazy; my doctor told me to get him out of my bed by the time he turned two months. I used to begrudge these needs, and occasionally still do when they conflict with my selfish wants. But this is a season, a hard season to be sure, but a relatively short one in the long run. It's not a perfect system, naps come late or end early if I can't be there for some reason, and it is one I have to continuously remind myself is best for baby even if it is hard for me. But the bottom line is I worked long and hard to conceive and create this life and I owe him the best of me. Right now that is my time and my presence, and I am going to make sure he gets all of it he wants.'*

'I spent six weeks trying to do 'the right thing', you know, put bub down semi-awake, swaddled, in her bassinet and pat her to sleep. It was stressful. We were just fighting one another and getting nowhere. At six weeks I thought enough is enough, I'll follow your lead. I starting feeding to sleep and co-sleeping in the mornings. Sleep and going to bed became a peaceful time, there are now no tears and our bond is amazing.'

'At eight months we tried a sleep consultant as my baby girl was waking every one to two hours. She assured us her techniques were 'emotionally supportive', but by three or four sessions in she was asking us to put her in her cot, leave her crying and sit nearby, saying soothing things. We didn't even get a minute or two in before we both had the sudden realisation that we would rather co-sleep and wake every hour for the next however many months than let her cry alone in her cot. Sometimes at night she wants us. We will always, always be there for her. Now at night we cuddle her just that little bit longer each night.'

'I'm a planner. I had a nursery kitted out and a crib ready in our room. When our baby arrived she fed a lot and cried whenever we put her down. After a few days taking it in turns sleeping, and starting to have hallucinations, we knew something had to change. We asked for help from family and clinicians and tried everything! We put her in a carrycot, we raised one end, we lay a hot water bottle down first and we padded the sides with towels. Nothing worked. After turning to Google my husband found information on safe bed-sharing on the internet. Further research convinced me sleeping this way was actually safer and beneficial in terms of emotional well-being, cognitive development and bonding. I felt a little angry at all of the misinformation! My little girl still wakes every two to four hours to feed, but rarely cries and is incredibly happy. Others told me to do controlled crying, or that I was spoiling her, but doing otherwise felt wrong and I felt was based on outdated research. We babywear for every nap as it's the only way she'll sleep. I was criticised a lot for that but it works for us and I can tell by how she will happily play by herself in our presence that she can do so as she feels so secure. I cope with the tiredness by going to bed when she does at half past seven at night and I know if I didn't bed-share I'd never have the energy to respond to her needs overnight.'

'We tried the bassinet by the bed when our daughter was very young and didn't understand what the struggle was about. It became a matter of biology for me when I would see my daughter immediately relaxed and contented when she slept on my chest. She slept on my chest for nearly five months until she felt more comfortable sleeping on a mattress on the floor next to me. My mother and some older relatives looked genuinely terrified when I told them I co-slept with her and tried to get me to sleep-train her immediately. Breastfeeding on demand, wearing her to sleep and co-sleeping all came so naturally for us and have made us such an intricately bonded pair. I do not claim to follow any official guidelines of 'attachment parenting', I simply follow my instincts. There is no way I can let her cry it out when every fibre of my being hates when she cries. My advice is to follow your instincts. We are biologically designed to respond quickly to our infants' cries. Once I figured that out I let go of the unwarranted parental advice I had been receiving from people who believe I spoil my baby.'

'Our daughter is two and a half years old now; we still nurse to sleep at night and co-sleep. We are the only parents we know not to have sleep-trained our baby. In the early newborn days I felt quite overwhelmed by all of the advice to 'put her down', 'get her settled in her Moses basket' and 'not carry her around because I was building bad habits'. I felt that she wanted to be held. She slept so peacefully next to me, but woke every 45 minutes alone. I felt she just wanted to be with mummy. As a first-time mum I didn't feel confident to follow my instincts, so instead started to read and came across gentle parenting and the research associated with it. It simply confirmed what I was feeling. It made sense. I think sometimes we forget what a huge transition it is to go from the lovely safe mummy womb to the outside world. I often think if we had the same transition in adulthood, we'd be in therapy for years! We expect so much of our little babies, to sleep alone when only days before they were inside us. So the main thing I've learnt is to trust my instincts; our babies were part of us, growing in our bodies; our bodies were doing the mummying without us thinking about it. We were mummies before we knew we were! So I try my best to follow my instincts. As a parent, if it feels wrong, somewhere in me is saying 'no no no', then for me, chances are it is wrong for me and my baby girl. Learning about gentle parenting has given me confidence. And now I can see my beautiful baby girl developing into a loving, brave and independent little girl, and I'm convinced it's because we've given her the security of responsiveness and attentiveness. Trust yourself. No one is more qualified, more experienced, more knowledgeable than you to respond to your baby.'

'After having my daughter, I felt none of the rush of emotions of love; in fact I felt nothing. When I got home, tired from birth and problems with breastfeeding due to tongue-tie, I found my feelings were even less for her. I felt nothing for her, she was more of a stress to me. Even a walk to the town which is five minutes from my home made me want to burst into tears. I was later diagnosed with PND. I was given endless advice from well-meaning friends and family to leave her to cry to let me 'have a break', and to 'teach her to be independent'. Even though I felt very little for her, I did feel this was wrong for us and I knew she needed me, regardless of my feelings. I recalled watching a television show years before with women carrying their babies in a sling. So I bought one to try. The first day I put her in, it was a like a release of some of the stress I was feeling. She didn't cry, she just went to sleep while I did the dishes. I then started to wear her in it all the time to sleep during the day. I believe it gave me the rest I needed from her as my hands were free to do what I wanted, while she got the closeness she wanted and needed. Now when I wear her, I love the feel of her close to me. Wearing her while she slept was truly healing for me, and even as a toddler she still loves it and gets a grin on her face when she sees one of our slings.'

'I am a 38-year-old first-time mum of a little girl conceived by IVF who is now six months old. I lost my own mum four years ago and I miss her advice. I was given parenting books for

Christmas, which I read while I was still pregnant. Although I didn't really take notice of any sleep-training content, my expectation became that our baby would sleep in the Moses basket in our room until six months then would go next door in her own room. Co-sleeping was a definite no no! I would deal with night waking as I intended to breastfeed and it would allow my partner to get sleep for work. My baby was induced at 38 weeks and I delivered her in only six hours and 45 minutes. The first night at home I kept her in bed all night to try and feed, which terrified my partner but felt strangely natural for me. For the first three weeks while my partner was on leave we were both waking to feed her and my partner would then rock her to sleep and place her in the Moses basket. After 23 nights of this and very little sleep I took her into bed with me after a two-hour crying session trying to rock her to sleep. Since that night we've never looked back. I set up our room with a sidecar cot and I now feed her to sleep every night. I took her to an osteopath who diagnosed and treated tensions in her cranium. She quietly wakes me in the night for feeds (two to four per night) and her dad doesn't hear a thing! She is not going into her own room any time soon. During the day she naps on me, with me on the bed or walking in her buggy or sling. I have had lots of comments about all of this but now I'm confident to argue my case if I care to, but I mostly ignore others' views and carry on with what works for us.'

'With our first child, now three years old, we followed all of the mainstream parenting advice, even though a lot was against our instincts. Into own room by about twelve weeks, sleep-trained at seventeen weeks, etc. The stress and guilt had always stayed with me, so second time around we are parenting differently. The baby sleeps beside me in our super-king bed with my husband the other side of me. I now know that night-waking

is normal, as is night-time parenting! He does not have his own cot and we have no intention of moving him out of our bed. It's also so much easier to feed him. I latch him on when he stirs and we both drift off to sleep. Breastfeeding has a rather lovely-sleep inducing effect on us both and its soooooo much easier than making up a bottle! He feeds fairly frequently, but it's for comfort as well as nutrition and I'm surprised to say that I don't really feel tired. I think I found it harder and more tiring sitting up to feed my first baby in a dark room and putting him back in his cot! Sleep training with my first baby caused me much anxiety and guilt; it's not worth going there and I now realise how stressful it will have been for him too. The fact he stopped crying and went to sleep is because he gave up hope that his caregivers would respond to him. Why do that to a child?'

'My first-born is now three and a half years old. When she was a baby I was aware of gentle sleep methods but I doubted my instincts. I obsessed about night-wakings, how long she'd napped for and worried that I was making a rod for my own back by carrying her in the sling for naps. It was the main topic of conversation with other mums. Our second-born is three months old. I'm pretty sure he sleeps and wakes in the night similarly to his sister but I feel so much more relaxed, happy and rested. I couldn't tell you how many times he woke to feed last night. I happily bed share and he goes straight back off to sleep after I feed him. All I ask myself in the morning is 'How do you feel today?' And generally I feel OK. I'm sure I feel this way due to not obsessing about sleep and understanding it's normal for babies to wake frequently. I'm so glad I now trust my instincts, I just wish I had done so more with our daughter. When you know better, you do better.'

'I feel that breastfeeding my daughter helped with my sleep post birth and even now at seven months. Breastfeeding meant I didn't have to get up during the night and make up bottles. Although it meant I was the only person who could feed her, I feel I got more sleep this way. My daughter would wake up, feed and settle and then go back down to sleep. The whole process took around 40 minutes. Then I could get back to sleep myself. Because of hormones released during feeding this aided me dropping back off to sleep. Also as my daughter fed to sleep as a small baby and even now at seven months for her bedtime feed it has always been a pretty certain way to get her to go to sleep.'

'Hands up – I'm a lazy, selfish mother! Or I was at the start. Most of my parenting decisions were initially made to make my life easier. We co-slept because it was easier and we both got more sleep. I wore him in a sling almost all the time, because he was much, much happier there and so my life was quieter and easier. The sound of a baby crying is like nails on a blackboard. I can't stand it. This is by design, apparently. They're not designed to be ignored. So to start with, my parenting decisions were purely selfish. But then... It turns out staying close to his perfect squishy little face wasn't a hardship at all. Being apart at night felt wrong. It went against every fibre of my being to put him down, or let him fuss a while, so I stopped listening to the people who told me I should. I've never believed that babies can be spoiled. No rods were made for my own back. The best piece of parenting advice I ever received was: 'Parent the child you have now'. Respond to their needs now without worrying what it might lead to. My perfect squishy boy moved into his own room at eleven months, without issue. He learned to settle himself at night, without issue. I have no idea if it's because we co-slept in the early days, or because I wore him all the time and never left him to cry. I do know that I enjoyed *his baby days far more than friends who were trying method after method to get their child to sleep through before they were biologically able, and who tried to put their babies down to get stuff done. I cooked, cleaned and pooed with the dude. No stress.'*

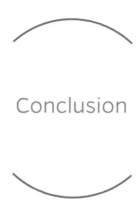

Conclusion

At the very beginning of this book I posed three questions:

- Why does baby sleep matter?
- Is it possible to meet the needs of both baby and parent?
- What happens when we do not respond to a baby's physical and psychological needs?

I would like to close by reconsidering them.

Why does baby sleep matter? It matters because it constitutes at least 50 per cent of the time we spend with our babies. If we are to raise confident, happy and independent adults, we must consider the effects of all of their earliest moments. We cannot realistically expect to create an individual who trusts others and believes that they are worthy of respect if we are not there for them at the times when they need us most as babies. We cannot expect them to respect themselves and others if they were not afforded that respect in their early days, weeks and months. This is what happens when we do not respond to a baby's physical and emotional needs at night. This is what we risk when we resort to mainstream 'cry-based' sleep-training. This is what we risk when we force separation of mother and infant.

Is it possible to meet the needs of both baby and parent? Yes, it is. Often, however, the 'answer' requires a hard look at how we live our own lives. A degree of introspection and self-questioning is required. What are we willing to sacrifice in order to meet the needs of our babies? What is really essential? How can we change our lives to enable us to meet the needs of our babies, by day and night, for what is really such a short time?

What is ultimately needed is a shift in our society's view of infant sleep. We must stop seeing babies' sleep as a 'problem' needing to be fixed, or an inconvenience that can be trained away. We must help parents to understand that normal baby sleep is not what they read in a magazine or see on television. We need to support families more – financially, physically and emotionally – so that they can parent in the way that is most natural and indeed most beneficial to our species. We need to create a movement to muffle the loud voice of the 'baby trainer', and to infiltrate as many sources of information as possible so that they are truly evidence-based. Our medical professionals desperately need better up-to-date education about infant sleep. Above all, though, we need to trust in our babies and in our instincts. If all we did was to follow our babies' lead and trust in ourselves, baby sleep problems would not exist at all.

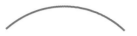

References

Chapter 1

1. Kopp, C.B., 'Antecedents of self-regulation: A developmental view', *Developmental Psychology*, 18, (1982), pp. 199-214.

2. Suchecki, D., Rosenfeld, P., Levine, S., 'Maternal regulation of the hypothalamic-pituitary-adrenal axis in the infant rat: the roles of feeding and stroking', *Developmental Brain Research,* Oct 15;75, (1993), pp. 185-92.

3. Flinn, M.V., Nepomnaschy, P.A., Muehlenbein, M.P., Ponzi, D., 'Evolutionary functions of early social modulation of hypothalamic–pituitary–adrenal axis development in humans', *Neuroscience and Biobehavioral Reviews*, 35 (7), (2011), pp. 1611–29.

4. Middlemiss, W., Granger, D.A., Goldberg, W.A., Nathans, L., 'Asynchrony of mother-infant hypothalamic-pituitary-adrenal axis activity following extinction of infant crying responses induced during the transition to sleep', *Early Human Development*, Apr;88(4), (2012), pp. 227-32.

5. Luby, J.L., Barch, D.M., Belden, A., Gaffrey, M.S., Tillman, R., Babb, C., Nishino, T., Suzuki, H., Botteron, K.N., 'Maternal support in early childhood predicts larger hippocampal volumes at school age', *Proceedings of the National Academy of Sciences*, 21;109(8), (2012), pp. 2854-9.

6. Spinrad, T.L., Stifter, C.A., Donelan-McCall, N., Turner, L. 'Mothers' regulation strategies in response to toddlers' affect: Links to later emotion self-regulation', *Social Development*, 13(1), (2004), pp. 40-55.

7. Kogan, N., & Carter, A., 'Mother-infant reengagement following the still-face: The role of maternal emotional availability in infant affect regulation', *Infant Behavior and Development*, 19, (1995), pp. 359-369.

Chapter 2

1. Graven, S.N., Browne, J.V., 'Sleep and Brain Development The Critical Role of Sleep in Fetal and Early Neonatal Brain Development', *Newborn and Infant Nursing Reviews*, Volume 8, Issue 4, (2008), pp. 173-179.
2. Roffwarg, H.P., Muzic, J.N., Dement, W.C., 'Ontogenetic development of the human sleep-dream cycle', *Science*, 7;152, (1966), pp. 604-619.
3. Bonmati-Carrion, M.A., Arguelles-Prieto, R., Martinez-Madrid, M.J., Reiter, R., Hardeland, R., Rol, M.A., Madrid, J.A., 'Protecting the melatonin rhythm through circadian healthy light exposure', *International Journal of Molecular Sciences*, (2014), Dec 17;15 (12), pp. 448-500.
4. Vartanian, G.V., Li, B.Y., Chervenak, A.P., Walch, O.J., Pack, W., Ala-Laurila, P., Wong, K.Y., 'Melatonin Suppression by Light in Humans Is More Sensitive Than Previously Reported', *Journal Biological Rhythms*, Aug;30(4), (2015), pp. 351-4.
5. Silva, M.L., Mallozi, M.C., Ferrari, G.F., 'Salivary cortisol to assess the hypothalamic-pituitary-adrenal axis in healthy children under 3 years old', *Journal Pediatrics*, Mar-Apr;83(2), (2007), pp. 121-6.
6. Joseph, D., Chong, N.W., Shanks, M.E., Rosato, E., Taub, N.A., Petersen, S.A., Symonds, M.E., Whitehouse, W.P., Wailoo, M., 'Getting rhythm: how do babies do it?', *Archives of Diseases of Childhood, Fetal Neonatal Edition*, Jan;100(1), (2015), pp. 50-4.
7. See www.history.vt.edu/Ekirch/sleepcommentary.html
8. Scammon, R.E., Doyle, L.O., 'Observations on the capacity of the stomach in the first ten days of postnatal life', *American Journal of Diseases of Children*, 20, (1920), pp. 516-538.
9. Wang, Y., 'Preliminary Study on the Blood Glucose Level in the Exclusively Breastfed Newborn', *Journal of Tropical Pediatrics*, 40, (1994), pp. 187-88.
10. Hirshkowitz, M., 'The National Sleep Foundation's Sleep Time Duration Recommendations: Results and Methodology Summary', *Sleep Health*, (2015).
11. Price, A.M.H., Quach, J., Wake, M., Bittman, M., Hiscock, H., 'Cross-sectional sleep thresholds for optimal health and wellbeing in Australian 4-9-year-olds', *Sleep Medicine*, published online: August 27, 2015
12. Anuntaseree, W., Mo-suwan, L., Vasiknanonte, P., Kuasirikul, S., Ma-

a-lee, A., Choprapawan. C., 'Night waking in Thai infants at 3 months of age: association between parental practices and infant sleep', *Sleep Medicine*, Jul;9(5), (2008), pp. 564-71.

13. Sadler, S., 'Sleep: what is normal at six months?', *Professional Care of Mother and Child*. Aug-Sep;4(6), (1994), pp.166-7.

14. Goodlin-Jones, B.L., Burnham, M.M., Gaylor, E.E., Anders, T.F., 'Night waking, sleep-wake organization, and self-soothing in the first year of life', *Journal Developmental Behavioural Pediatrics*, Aug;22(4), (2001), pp. 226-33.

15. Hall, W.A., Liva, S., Moynihan, M., Saunders, R., 'A comparison of actigraphy and sleep diaries for infants' sleep behavior', *Frontiers in Psychiatry*, Feb 12, (2015), pp. 6-19.

Chapter 3

1. Seehagen, S., Konrad, C., Herbert, J.S., 'Timely sleep facilitates declarative memory consolidation in infants', *Proceedings of the National Academy of Sciences*, published online 12 January 2015

2. LeBourgeois, M.K1., Carskadon, M.A., Akacem, L.D., Simpkin, C.T., Wright, K.P. Jr., Achermann, P., Jenni, O.G., 'Circadian phase and its relationship to nighttime sleep in toddlers', *Journal of Biological Rhythms*, Oct;28(5), (2013), pp. 322-31.

3. Iglowstein, I., Jenni, O.G., Molinari, L., Largo, R.H., 'Sleep duration from infancy to adolescence: Reference values and generational trends', *Pediatrics*,111(2), (2003), pp. 302-307.

4. Thorpe, K., Staton, S., Sawyer, E., Pattinson, C., Haden, C., Smith, C., 'Napping, development and health from 0 to 5 years: a systematic review', *Archives of Disease in Childhood*, 100, (2015), pp. 615-622.

5. Hunziker, U.A., Barr, R.G., 'Increased carrying reduces infant crying: a randomized controlled trial', *Pediatrics*. May;77(5), (1986), pp. 641-8.

6. Blair, P.S., Ward Platt, M.W., Smith, I.J., Fleming, P.J., 'Sudden Infant Death Syndrome and the time of death', *International Journal of Epidemiology*, 35 (6), (2006), pp. 1563-1569.

7. Chellappa, S.L., Steiner, R., Oelhafen, P., Lang, D., Götz, T., Krebs, J., Cajochen, C., 'Acute exposure to evening blue-enriched light impacts on human sleep', *Journal of Sleep Research*, Oct;22(5), (2013), pp. 573-80.

8. Smolensky, M.H., Sackett-Lundeen, L.L., Portaluppi, F., 'Nocturnal light pollution and underexposure to daytime sunlight: Complementary mechanisms of circadian disruption and related diseases', *Chronobiology International*, Sep 16:1-20 (2015), pp. 1029-48.

9. Tsai, S.Y., Thomas, K.A., Lentz, M.J., Barnard KE., 'Light is beneficial for

infant circadian entrainment: an actigraphic study', *Journal of Advanced Nursing*, Aug;68(8), (2012), pp. 1738-47.

Chapter 4

1. Jenness, R., 'The composition of human milk', *Seminars in Perinatology*, Jul;3(3), (1979), pp. 225-39.

2. Tay, C.C., Glasier, A.F., McNeilly, A.S., 'Twenty-four hour patterns of prolactin secretion during lactation and the relationship to suckling and the resumption of fertility in breast-feeding women', *Human Reproduction*, May;11(5), (1996), pp. 950-5.

3. Cohen Engler, A., Hadash, A., Shehadeh, N., Pillar, G., 'Breastfeeding may improve nocturnal sleep and reduce infantile colic: potential role of breast milk melatonin', *European Journal of Pediatrics*, Apr;171(4), (2012), pp. 729-32.

4. Goldman, A. S., 'The immune system of human milk: Antimicrobial anti-inflammatory and immunomodulating properties', *Pediatric Infectious Disease Journal*, 12(8), (1993), pp. 664-671.

5. Sánchez, C.L., Cubero, J., Sánchez, J., 'The possible role of human milk nucleotides as sleep inducers', *Nutritional Neuroscience*, 12, (2009), pp. 2–8.

6. Carver, J.D., 'Advances in nutritional modifications of infant formulas', *American Journal of Clinical Nutrition*, vol. 77 (6), (2003), pp. 1550-1554.

7. Cubero, J., Narciso, D., Terrón, P., Rial, R., Esteban, S., Rivero, M., Parvez, H., Rodríguez, A.B., Barriga, C., 'Chrononutrition applied to formula milks to consolidate infants' sleep/wake cycle', *Neuro Endocrinology Letters*, 2007 Aug;28(4), (2007), pp. 360-6.

8. Doan, T., Gay, C.L., Kennedy, H.P., Newman, J., Lee, K.A., 'Nighttime breastfeeding behavior is associated with more nocturnal sleep among first-time mothers at one month postpartum', *Journal of Clinical Sleep Medicine*. Mar 15;10(3), (2014), pp. 313-9.

9. Cohen Engler, A., Hadash, A., Shehadeh, N., Pillar, G., 'Breastfeeding may improve nocturnal sleep and reduce infantile colic: potential role of breast milk melatonin', *European Journal of Pediatrics*, Apr;171(4), (2012), pp. 729-32.

10. Cubero, J., Valero, V., Sánchez, J., Rivero, M., Parvez, H., Rodríguez, A.B., Barriga, C., 'The circadian rhythm of tryptophan in breast milk affects the rhythms of 6-sulfatoxymelatonin and sleep in newborn', *Neuro Endocrinology Letters*, Dec;26(6), (2005), pp. 657-61.

11. Tu, M.T., Lupien, S.J., Walker, C.D., 'Diurnal Salivary Cortisol Levels In Postpartum Mothers As A Function Of Infant Feeding Choice And

Parity', *Psychoneuroendocrinology*, Aug;31(7), (2006), pp. 812-24.

12. Figueiredo, B., Dias, C.C., Brandão, S., Canário, C., Nunes-Costa, R., 'Breastfeeding and postpartum depression: state of the art review', *Journal of Pediatrics*, Jul-Aug;89(4), (2013), pp. 332-8.

Chapter 5

1. Brown, A., Harries, V., 'Infant sleep and night feeding patterns during later infancy', *Breastfeeding Medicine*, June, 10(5), (2015), pp. 246-252.

2. Macknin, M.L., Medendorp, S.V., Maier, M.C., 'Infant sleep and bedtime cereal', *American Journal Diseases of Children*, Sep;143(9), (1989), pp. 1066-8

3. Keane, V., 'Do solids help baby sleep through the night?', *American Journal of Diseases of Children*, 142, (1988), pp. 404-05.

Chapter 7

1. Yang, C.K., Hahn, H.M., 'Cosleeping in young Korean children', *Journal of Developmental and Behavioural Pediatrics*, Jun;23(3), (2002), pp.151-7.

2. Latz, S., Wolf, A.W., Lozoff, B., 'Cosleeping in context: sleep practices and problems in young children in Japan and the United States', *Archives Pediatric Adolescent Medicine*, Apr;153(4), (1999), pp. 339-46.

3. Worthman, C.M., Brown, R.A., 'Companionable sleep: social regulation of sleep and cosleeping in Egyptian families', *Journal Family Psychology*, Mar;21(1), (2007), pp. 124-35.

4. Mindell, J.A., Sadeh, A., Wiegand, B., How, T.H., Goh, D.Y., 'Cross-cultural differences in infant and toddler sleep', *Sleep Medicine*, Mar;11(3), (2010), pp. 274-80.

5. Mindell, J.A., Sadeh. A., Kwon, R., Goh, D.Y., 'Cross-cultural comparison of maternal sleep', *Sleep*, Nov 1;36(11), (2013), pp. 1699-706.

6. Barry, H., Paxson, L.M., 'Infancy and Early Childhood: Cross Cultural Codes', *Ethnology*, 10, (1971), pp. 466-508.
7. Whiting, E., 'Culture and Human Development: The Selected Papers of John Whiting', *Cambridge University Press,* New edition (2006).

8. Morelli, G.A., Rogoff, B., Oppenheim, D., Goldsmith, D., 'Cultural Variation in Infants' Sleeping Arrangements: Questions of Independence', *Developmental Psychology*, Vol 28, no.4, (1992), pp. 604-613.

9. LeBourgeois, M.K., Carskadon, M.A., Akacem, L.D., Simpkin, C.T., Wright, K.P., Achermann, P., Jenni, O.G., 'Circadian phase and its relationship to nighttime sleep in toddlers', *Journal Biologicial Rhythms*, Oct;28(5), (2013), pp. 322-31.

Chapter 8

1. Ball, H.L., 'Reasons to bed-share: why parents sleep with their infants', *Journal of Reproductive and Infant Psychology*, 20(4), (2002), pp. 207-222.

2. Bolling, K., Grant, C., Hamlyn, B., 'Infant Feeding Survey 2005', *The Information Centre for Health and Social Care*, 2007.

3. Ateah, C.A, Hamelin, K.J., 'Maternal bedsharing practices, experiences, and awareness of risks', *Journal of Obstetric, Gynecologic, and Neonatal Nursing*, 37(3), (2008), pp. 274-81.

4. Lahr, M.B., Rosenberg, K.D., Lapidus, J.A., 'Bedsharing and maternal smoking in a population-based survey of new mothers', *Pediatrics*, Oct;116(4), (2005), pp. 530-42.

5. Nelson, E.A., Chan, P.H., 'Child care practices and cot death in Hong Kong', *New Zealand Medical Journal*,1996 Apr 26;109(1020), (1996), pp. 144-6.

6. Fukumizu, M., Kaga, M., Kohyama, J., Hayes, M.J., 'Sleep-related nighttime crying (yonaki) in Japan: a community-based study', *Pediatrics*, Jan;115(2005), pp. 217-24.

7. Mindell, J.A., Sadeh, A., Kohyama, J., How, T.H., 'Parental behaviors and sleep outcomes in infants and toddlers: a cross-cultural comparison', *Sleep Medicine*, Apr;11(4), (2010), pp. 393-9.

8. Willinger, M., Ko, C.W., Hoffman, H.J., Kessler, R.C., Corwin, M.J., 'National Infant Sleep Position study. Trends in infant bed sharing in the United States, 1993-2000: the National Infant Sleep Position study', *Archives Pediatric Adolescent Medicine*, Jan;157(1), (2003), pp. 43-9.

9. Wert, K.M., Lindemeyer, R., Spatz, D.L., 'Breastfeeding, co-sleeping and dental health advice', *American Journal Maternity and Child Nursing*, May-Jun;40(3), (2015), pp. 174-9.

10. McKenna, J.J., Gettler, L.T., 'There is no such thing as infant sleep, there is no such thing as breastfeeding, there is only breastsleeping', *Acta Paediatrica*, Aug 21 (2015), doi: 10.1111/apa.13161. [Epub ahead of print].

11. Vennemann, M.M., Bajanowski, T., Brinkmann, B., Jorch, G., Yücesan, K., Sauerland, C., Mitchell, E.A., 'Does Breastfeeding Reduce the Risk of Sudden Infant Death Syndrome?', *Pediatrics*, Vol. 123(3), (2009), pp.406-410.

12. Ball, H.L., 'Breastfeeding, bed-sharing, and infant sleep', *Birth*, 30(3), (2003), pp. 181-8.

13. McCoy, R.C., Hunt, C.E., Lesko, S.M., 'Frequency of bed sharing and its relationship to breastfeeding', *Journal of Developmental and Behavioural*

Pediatrics, 25(3), (2004), pp. 141-9.

14. Blair, P.S., Heron, J., Fleming, P.J., 'Relationship between bed sharing and breastfeeding: longitudinal, population-based analysis', *Pediatrics*, Nov;126(5), (2010), pp. 1119-26.

15. Academy of Breastfeeding Medicine, 'Cosleeping and Breastfeeding Academy Breastfeeding Medicine, Protocol', http://www.bfmed.org/Resources/Protocols.aspx, accessed online 20/10/2015,

16. Blair, P. S., 'Bed-Sharing in the Absence of Hazardous Circumstances: Is There a Risk of Sudden Infant Death Syndrome? An Analysis from Two Case-Control Studies Conducted in the UK', *PLoS One*, September 19;9(9), (2014).

17. UNICEF statement on draft NICE Co-sleeping Guidelines. http://www.unicef.org.uk/BabyFriendly/News-and-Research/News/UNICEF-UK-statement-on-draft-NICE-guidelines-on-co-sleeping-and-SIDS/. Accessed online 20/10/2015.

18. Baddock, S.A., Galland, B.C., Beckers, M.G., Taylor, B.J., Bolton. D.P., 'Bed-sharing and the infant's thermal environment in the home setting', *Archives Diseases of Childhood*, Dec;89(12) (2004), pp. 1111-6.

19. Ball, H., 'Airway covering during bed-sharing', *Child Care Health Development*, Sep;35(5), (2009), pp. 728-37.

20. Baddock, S.A., Galland, B.C., Bolton, D.P., Williams, S.M., Taylor, B.J., 'Differences in infant and parent behaviors during routine bed sharing compared with cot sleeping in the home setting', *Pediatrics*, May;117(5), (2006). pp. 1599-607.

21. Gettler, L.T., McKenna, J.J., McDade, T.W., Agustin, S.S., Kuzawa, C.W., 'Does cosleeping contribute to lower testosterone levels in fathers? Evidence from the Philippines,' *PLoS One*, 7(9), (2012).

22. Beijers, R., Riksen-Walraven, J.M., de Weerth, C., 'Cortisol regulation in 12-month-old human infants: associations with the infants' early history of breastfeeding and co-sleeping', *Stress*, 2013 May;16(3), (2013), pp. 267-77.

23. Olsen, N.J., Buch-Andersen, T., Händel, M.N., Ostergaard, L.M., Pedersen, J., Seeger, C., Stougaard, M., Trærup, M., Livemore, K., Mortensen, E.L., Holst, C., Heitmann, B.L., 'The Healthy Start project: a randomized, controlled intervention to prevent overweight among normal weight, preschool children at high risk of future overweight', *BMC Public Health*, Aug 1;12, (2012), pp. 590.

24. Okami, P., Weisner, T., Olmstead, R., 'Outcome correlates of parent-child bedsharing: an eighteen-year longitudinal study', *Journal of Developmental and Behavioural Pediatrics*, Aug;23(4), (2002), pp. 244-53.

25. Mosko, S., Richard, C., McKenna, J., Drummond, S., Mukai, D., 'Maternal proximity and infant CO2 environment during bedsharing and possible implications for SIDS research', *American Journal of Physical Anthropology*, Jul;103(3), (1997), pp. 315-28.

Chapter 9

1. Garcia, A.J., Koschnitzky, J.E., Ramirez, J.M., 'The physiological determinants of Sudden Infant Death Syndrome', *Respiratory Physiology and Neurobiology*, 189(2), (2013), pp. 288-300.

2. Randall, B.B., Paterson, D.S., Haas, E.A., Broadbelt, K.G., Duncan, J.R., Mena, O.J., Krous, H.F., Trachtenberg, F.L., Kinney, H.C., 'Potential asphyxia and brainstem abnormalities in sudden and unexpected death in infants', *Pediatrics*, 132(6), (2013), pp.1616-25.

3. Fleming, P., Blair, P.S., 'Sudden Infant Death Syndrome and parental smoking', *Early Human Development*, 83, (2007), pp. 721-725.

4. Blair, P.S., Fleming, P.J., Smith, I.J., 'Babies sleeping with parents: case-control study of factors influencing the risk of the sudden infant death syndrome', *BMJ*, 319(7223), (1999), pp. 1457–1462

5. Carpenter, R.G., Irgens, L.M., Blair, P.S., England, P.D., Fleming, P., Huber, J., 'Sudden unexplained infant death in 20 regions in Europe: case control study', *Lancet*, 363(9404), (2004), pp. 185-91.

6. McVea, K.L., Turner, P.D., Peppler, D.K., 'The role of breastfeeding in sudden infant death syndrome', *Journal of Human Lactation*, 16(1), (2000), pp.13-20.

7. Hauck, F.R., Herman, S.M., Donovan, M., 'Sleep environment and the risk of sudden infant death syndrome in an urban population: the Chicago Infant Mortality Study', *Pediatrics*, 111(5 pt 2), (2003), pp. 1207–1214.

8. Bergman, N.J., 'Proposal for mechanisms of protection of supine sleep against sudden infant death syndrome: an integrated mechanism review', *Pediatric Research*, Jan;77(1-1), (2015), pp. 10-9.

9. Horne, R.S., Hauck, F.R., Moon, R.Y., L'hoir, M.P., Blair, P.S., 'Dummy (pacifier) use and sudden infant death syndrome: potential advantages and disadvantages', *Journal Paediatric Child Health*, 2014 Mar;50(3), (2014), pp. 170-4.

10. Downham, M.A., Stanton, A.N., 'Keep cool, baby: the risks of over-heating in young babies', *Health Visiting*, 54(8), (1981), pp. 325-8 104.

11. Bacon, C.J., 'Over heating in infancy', *Archives of Diseases in Childhood*, 58(9), (1983), pp. 673-4 105.

12. Stanton, A.N., 'Sudden infant death. Overheating and cot death', *Lancet*,

324(8413), (1984), pp.1199-201.

13. Williams, S.M., Taylor, B.J., Mitchell, E.A., 'Sudden infant death syndrome: insulation from bedding and clothing and its effect modifiers', *International Journal of Epidemiology*, 25(2), (1996), pp. 366-75.

14. Sauseng, W., Kerbl, R., Thaller, S., Hanzer, M., Zotter, H., 'Baby sleeping bag and conventional bedding conditions--comparative investigations by infrared thermography', *Klinische Pädiatrie*, Sep;223(5), (2011), pp. 276-9.

15. Blair, P.S., Sidebotham, P., Evason-Coombe, C., Edmonds, M., Heckstall-Smith, E.M., Fleming, P., 'Hazardous cosleeping environments and risk factors amenable to change: case-control study of SIDS in south west England', *BMJ*, Oct 13, (2009), pp. 339-66.

16. Kato, I., Franco, P., Groswasser, J., Scaillet, S., Kelmanson,I.A., Togari, H., 'Incomplete arousal processes in infants who were victims of sudden death', *American Journal of Respiratory Critical Care Medicine*, 168, (2003), pp. 1298–303.

17. Wilson, C.A., Taylor, B.J., Laing, R.M., Williams, S.M., Mitchell, E.A., 'Clothing and bedding and its relevance to sudden infant death syndrome: further results from the New Zealand Cot Death Study', *Journal Paediatric Child Health*, 30, (1994), pp. 506–12.

18. Ponsonby, A.L., Dwyer, T., Gibbons, L.E., Cochrane, J.A., Wang, Y.G., 'Factors potentiating the risk of sudden infant death syndrome associated with the prone position', *New England Journal of Medicine*, 329(6), (1993), pp. 377–82.

Chapter 11

1. Etebary, S., Nikseresht, S., Sadeghipour, H.R., Zarrindast, M.R., 'Postpartum Depression and Role of Serum Trace Elements', *Iranian Journal of Psychiatry*, Spring; 5(2), (2010), pp. 40–46.

2. Patel, R.R., Murphy, D.J., Peters, T.J., 'Operative delivery and postnatal depression: a cohort study', *BMJ*, April (16), (2005), pp. 330.

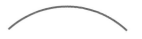

Further Reading and Resources

Books

La Leche League International, *Sweet Sleep: Nighttime and Naptime Strategies for the Breastfeeding Family*, 2014, Pinter & Martin.

McKenna, J., *Sleeping With Your Baby: A Parent's Guide to Co-Sleeping*, 2007, Platypus Media.

Middlemiss, W., Kendall-Tackett, K., *The Science of Mother-Infant Sleep: Current Findings on Bedsharing, Breastfeeding, Sleep Training and Normal Infant Sleep*, 2013, Praeclarus Press.

Ockwell-Smith, S., *The Gentle Sleep Book: A Guide for Calm Babies, Toddlers and Pre-Schoolers*, 2015, Piatkus.

Websites

Attachment Parenting International:
www.attachmentparenting.org
Attachment Parenting UK: www.attachmentparenting.co.uk
Evolutionary Parenting: www.evolutionaryparenting.com
Gentle Parenting: www.gentleparenting.co.uk

Infant Sleep Information Source (ISIS): www.isisonline.org.uk
Kellymom (Breastfeeding Information): www.kellymom.com
La Leche League International: www.llli.org
La Leche League UK: www.laleche.org.uk
Mother-Baby Behavioural Sleep Laboratory:
    www.cosleeping.nd.edu
The Lullaby Trust (formerly FSIDS): www.lullabytrust.org.
Sarah Ockwell-Smith's Blog: www.sarahockwell-smith.com

Social media

Evolutionary Parenting on Facebook: www.facebook.com/
    EvolutionaryParenting
Infant Sleep Information Source on Facebook: www.
    facebook.com/ISISonline
Pinter & Martin on Facebook: www.facebook.com/
    pinterandmartin
Sarah Ockwell-Smith on Facebook: www.facebook.com/
    sarahockwellsmithauthor
Sarah Ockwell-Smith on Twitter: www.twitter.com/
    TheBabyExpert
Why Your Baby's Sleep Matters on Facebook: www.facebook.
    com/Why-Your-Babys-Sleep-Matters

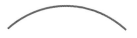

Acknowledgements

I would like to thank all of the wonderful parents from the 'Gentle Parenting UK' and 'Gentle Parenting International' Facebook discussion groups for their valuable contributions to this book. It wouldn't have been possible without you.

I would also like to thank any health professionals who may be reading this book. Your interest and dedication offers a much-needed ray of hope in a sea of outdated authoritarian sleep advice. On behalf of all of the new families that you will come into contact with over the years, a very big 'thank you' for wanting to turn the tide.

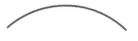

Index

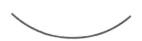